T0125771

TWIN

to

TWIN

PRAISE FOR
TWIN TO TWIN

"*An inspirational and heart-wrenching book.*"

—Cea Sunrise Person, author of bestselling memoir *North of Normal*

"*An 'orphan' disease, expectant mothers with Twin to Twin (and their support systems) should adopt Crystal Duffy's new memoir Twin to Twin. An intimate account, told with flagging and unflagging optimism, Duffy's story ensures that others need not ride alone through this rollercoaster experience.*"

—Suzy Becker, international bestselling author of *All I Need to Know I Learned from My Cat* and *One Good Egg*

"*Crystal Duffy's wit and self-deprecating humor helped her survive the realities and (sometimes devastating) physical and emotional truths of her high-stakes twin pregnancy. Twin to Twin is an engaging, compelling, and yes, entertaining read.*"

—Susan Krawitz, author of *Viva Rose*

"*Crystal's story is so moving and dramatic—the things that she, Ed, Abby, and her twins went through! She makes it all come alive with emotion and humor and honesty and pain, and I felt like I was right there with her.*"

—Jane Roper, author of *Double Time*

"*Imagine the worst day of your life so far, then multiply that by infinity. We imagine that is how Crystal Duffy must have felt the day she was told her twin pregnancy was threatened by twin to twin transfusion syndrome (TTTS). A potentially fatal disease that can take away one or both babies, TTTS is one of the least discussed issues in books about multiples—because it IS scary. Duffy dives bravely into her new frightening reality and emerges on the other side with a message of hope and optimism. Her must-read story is one of courage, honesty, family, and above all else, love.*"

—**Megan Woolsey** and **Alison Lee**, editors of *Multiples Illuminated: A Collection of Stories and Advice from Parents of Twins, Triplets and More* and the sequel *Multiples Illuminated: Life with Twins and Triplets, the Toddler to Tween Years*

"*An exciting ride through a delightful and surprising diagnosis that quickly turned terrifying. You'll empathize with Crystal, cheer for her, and draw strength for your own struggles.*"

—**Margaret Welwood**, author and mother of twins

"*Twin to Twin chronicles Crystal Duffy's journey through her high-risk, high-stakes twin pregnancy. Both beautiful and painful, the book, with glorious details and pacing, shows the power of one mother's love and resilience against all odds.*"

—**Marcelle Soviero**, Editor-in-Chief *Brain, Child: The Magazine for Thinking Mothers*

"*Twin to Twin is a compelling story of motherhood, told with passion, precision and power.*"

—**Marya Hornbacher**, *New York Times* bestselling author of *Wasted* and *Madness*

"*Crystal did great after such a complicated pregnancy.* Twin to Twin *is both an exciting and dramatic read that brings to life the fears and challenges of a high-risk pregnancy. This memoir is a powerful resource for parents, family members and friends, but also for professionals, including physicians, nurses, therapists and genetic counselors.*"

—Dr. Paul Cook, MD, with The OB/GYN Center of Houston affiliated with Children's Memorial Hermann Hospital

"Twin to Twin *is a riveting, poignant memoir about Crystal Duffy's turbulent journey through her high-risk pregnancy with identical twin daughters. With just the right amounts of self-reflection, humor, pathos, and joy, the author takes us through her harrowing diagnosis and in utero treatment of twin to twin transfusion syndrome. The book explores the many life sustaining connections that help Mrs. Duffy endure her separation from her twenty-two-month-old daughter while being hospitalized for five weeks to monitor the health of the two fetuses. This well written sensitive story is inspirational and spiritually uplifting. Mrs. Duffy's experiences compel the reader to celebrate the maternal courage, fortitude, and bravery needed to endure unforeseen emotional and physical complications related to childbearing.*"

—Joan A. Friedman, PhD, psychotherapist and author of *Emotionally Healthy Twins* and *Twins in Session: Case Histories in Treating Twin Issues*

"*Crystal's book makes you realize that while not every twin parenting moment is rosy, it does make you stronger, and many of the darkest moments can make you a better parent, and a better woman.*"

—Natalie Diaz, founder and CEO of Twiniversity and bestselling author of *What to Do When You're Having Two*

"I thoroughly enjoyed reading this book. It describes a mother's experience dealing with the ever-changing drama of twin pregnancy with complications. Duffy has written the account in such a way that anyone, whether the reader knows about the subject matter or not, they can relate to it in some way. It is charming, witty, at times sad but very uplifting description of human determination and resilience. As a physician who deals with the outcomes of such pregnancies and is always searching the best way to help mothers and families understand what to expect during such situations, this book will be an essential tool."

—Dr. Amir Khan, MD, Neonatal Perinatal Medicine Specialist, Memorial Hermann Texas Medical Center

"In her book, Twin to Twin, Crystal Duffy (who calls herself `feisty' and her pregnant body a `science project') shares her journey through loss, pregnancy, renewal, and the miracle of being part of the 1 percent of mothers with a Mono-Mono twin pregnancy. Buoyed by her faith, the love of her husband, Ed, and a cast of unlikely heroes at the hospital worthy of their own sitcom—like Paul, the male nurse she binge watches Bravo's Housewives shows with, and the music therapist, Charlotte, who helps her channel her suffering into song—Crystal shares every stage of her perilous journey toward birthing her babies, with honesty, humility and humor. Everyone has a birth story but this one will move you to tears, make you chuckle, and count your blessings along with Crystal as she illustrates, through words and poetry, her weeks as a hospital inpatient, and the path that led to her current work as an antepartum and neonatal patient advocate."

—Estelle Erasmus, journalist, writing coach, Writer's Digest University instructor, and host of ASJA Direct podcast

"Anyone in the field of fetal medicine, or any field of medicine for that matter, should consider reading Crystal's book. It is an uninhibited disclosure of a mother's experience with a life-threatening pregnancy complication. Not only does it show the sometimes yawning chasm between what doctor's counsel and what patients hear, but Crystal reveals it with clarity, wit, and empathy. Her story displays the extraordinary courage of a pregnant mother and the enduring compassion, talent, and wisdom of her team of providers. It is an uplifting example of what humans do best: care for each other. This book is Crystals way of caring by sharing her experience so that others can benefit."

—**Stephen P. Emery**, MD, Director, Center for Innovative Fetal Intervention, Magee-Women's Hospital of the University of Pittsburgh Medical Center (UPMC)

TWIN

to

TWIN

FROM HIGH-RISK PREGNANCY TO HAPPY FAMILY

Crystal Duffy

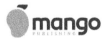

Mango Publishing

CORAL GABLES

Copyright © 2018 Crystal Duffy

Cover & Layout Design: Jermaine Lau

Mango is an active supporter of authors' rights to free speech and artistic expression in their books. The purpose of copyright is to encourage authors to produce exceptional works that enrich our culture and our open society. Uploading or distributing photos, scans or any content from this book without prior permission is theft of the author's intellectual property. Please honor the author's work as you would your own. Thank you in advance for respecting our authors' rights.

For permission requests, please contact the publisher at:

Mango Publishing Group
2850 Douglas Road, 3rd Floor
Coral Gables, FL 33134 USA
info@mango.bz

For special orders, quantity sales, course adoptions and corporate sales, please email the publisher at sales@mango.bz. For trade and wholesale sales, please contact Ingram Publisher Services at customer.service@ingramcontent.com or +1.800.509.4887.

Twin to Twin: From High-risk Pregnancy to Happy Family

Library of Congress Cataloging
ISBN: (print) 978-1-63353-833-7 (ebook) 978-1-63353-834-4

Library of Congress Control Number: 2018957578

BISAC category code: BIO026000
BIOGRAPHY & AUTHOBIOGRAPHY / Personal Memoirs

Printed in the United States of America

For Katherine and Lauren, my inspiration for it all.

For Abby and Ed, my strength through it all.

TABLE OF CONTENTS

AUTHOR'S NOTE

This is the story of my twin pregnancy. To write this book, I drew on
my personal journals, researched medical information and facts,
and consulted with several of the people who appear in the book. I
have changed the names of most, but not all, of the individuals in this
book, and in some cases, I also modified identifying details in order to
preserve anonymity. There are no composite characters or events in
the book. I occasionally omitted people and events, but only when that
omission had no impact or substance to the story.

FOREWORD

Having more than one baby in a pregnancy has always intrigued pregnant women. Perhaps it is considered a blessing by some to increase a family by two at one time. When I started my residency training in Obstetrics and Gynecology, I remember reading the phrase "the human womb is only designed to carry one fetus at a time with any degree of biological grace." Indeed, some forty years later, I have come to appreciate the truth in this statement. In those early years of my career, one in eighty pregnant women carried twins. The advent of assisted reproductive technologies (IVF and other methods) and a growing trend to defer motherhood until later in life have increased the incidence of twins to one in thirty pregnancies.

Once, all twin pregnancies were treated the same. Now, we know that identical or monochorionic (MC) twins can develop severe complications as often as four out of ten cases. This type of twinning is rare—only three out of 1000 pregnancies. It is a chance of nature, although the incidence is reported to be higher in IVF pregnancies. One of the complications of MC twins is severe twin-twin transfusion syndrome (TTTS)—this occurs in only 10 percent of these pregnancies. Shared blood vessels in the single placenta allow for blood movement between the patient's unborn babies—one becomes a "donor" and one a "recipient." Without treatment the loss of both twins occurs in 90 percent of cases. Some thirty years ago, in utero laser therapy was introduced to spot weld these connecting blood vessels using a small telescope (fetoscope) to find them in the womb. Although premature delivery remains an unsolved problem, experienced centers now report the survival of both twins in more than 70 percent of TTTS pregnancies.

In her book, Crystal tells the story of the highs and lows in her desire to have a successful pregnancy. She shares with the reader the sorrow of pregnancy loss and the elation of discovering that she had spontaneously conceived identical twins. Her joy is short-lived when she is diagnosed with TTTS. The reader is then taken down a journey of treatment, complications and the need for a prolonged stay in the hospital before she delivers her premature twin girls. The author's narrative is told in a unique first person perspective that allows the reader to look in on the emotions of separation from Crystal's husband and her first born daughter while she is hospitalized before delivery. Unique bonds are developed with the nursing staff, her obstetrician, and her sonographer. Crystal also shares the anxiety of separation from her newborn girls as they mature in the neonatal intensive care unit. The book concludes with a return to elation as the new family of five is finally reunited at home.

Medicine is a unique profession. A patient like Crystal meets you in the worst of circumstances, yet she is willing to place complete trust in your knowledge and skills to care for her unborn children. There can be no greater privilege than this. Since I learned to perform laser treatment fifteen years ago, I have undertaken over 700 procedures. Each case is unique. There have been many successes such as Crystal's pregnancy. And yet, there have been frustrating losses even when the procedure goes well from a technical point of view.

To be asked to author the introduction to this book is a unique honor. It truly tells the story of a patient's trials and tribulations with TTTS. The book is a must read for any patient diagnosed with TTTS. It will provide hope that all is not lost in their pregnancy.

John Moise

Kenneth J Moise Jr, MD (a.k.a. Dr. Miller)
Professor of Obstetrics, Gynecology and Reproductive Medicine
McGovern School of Medicine – UT Health
Co-Director, The Fetal Center
Children's Memorial Hermann Hospital
Houston, Texas

PART 1:

THE BEGINNING

THE ULTRASOUND

Certificates and degrees crowded the wall above a large wooden desk full of patient charts and scattered papers. The perinatologist seemed well-accredited, but not particularly neat. A trickle of natural light illuminated the mostly darkened room, let in by a folded-back corner of the blackout curtains over the room's sole window. The doctor specialized in high-risk pregnancies, and the ultrasound he was about to give me could forever change the course of mine. Or, it could be just another routine scan and all would be the same as it was before.

My mom, dad, and two-year-old daughter, Abby, were in the exam room with me. They were seated on a black upholstered couch angled in such a way that they could view the large ultrasound screen on the opposite wall. My dad's sneakers tapped on the linoleum floor. Abby lay on her stomach, her elbows pressed up against my mom. She kicked her legs gently back and forth. She giggled as she held up the screen to her iPad while she watched *Curious George*.

There was a brisk knock on the door and a nurse, a petite brunette in her mid-twenties, entered. She asked me to lie back on the exam table. The paper crinkled loudly beneath me as I struggled to find a comfortable position—a nearly impossible task for a twenty-three week pregnant woman with twins. A few days before, the everyday discomfort of gestating two babies had taken a sharp, dangerous turn. I was suddenly in agony, an intense pain that I had not been able to fully articulate to Dr. Cooper, my OB. Painful spasms were shooting down my spinal cord, and I'd started to feel a continuous sensation of a hard, tightened abdomen. I was suddenly expanding rapidly—and it wasn't just in my mind. I recalled the previous week's conversation with

Dr. Cooper during a routine visit; as I stood on his scale, it showed me I'd gained eight pounds in a mere week. "Are you kidding me?" I said to him. "How is this possible?" I felt like Violet, the rude girl in Charlie in the Chocolate Factory who inflates hugely after she chews the forbidden Wonka gum—like I would burst at any moment.

The nurse wrapped the cuff around my arm and took my blood pressure, scribbled the numbers in my chart. "This might be a little cold," she said as she pulled up my blouse. She grabbed a small white tube of ultrasound gel and began to rub it all over my belly. Her touch was soothing. It reminded me how I missed having massages at the spa. *After I have the babies, I'll have to book myself an appointment,* I thought.

My massage was interrupted by a knock on the door. I sat up instinctively, dripping some of the gel onto the top of my shorts. "All right, Crystal," said the perinatologist, as he walked into the exam room. A soft-spoken man with warm brown eyes, salt and pepper hair, and a red polka dot bow tie under his starched white lab coat; he bore a strong resemblance to Bill Nye the Science Guy. "Let's have a look at these babies," he said.

I nodded my head fiercely and leaned slowly back on the examining table. "Okay," I croaked as I adjusted my shorts. My heart was pounding so fast I wondered if anyone could hear it. No doubt my babies could as they were kicking up a storm, probably telling me to chill out.

Dr. Bill Nye sat down on his medical stool, grabbed the wand and began sliding it across my belly. He scanned silently for a few seconds. Then he leaned in close to the monitor and glided the wand back to the other side. He bit his bottom lip, steadied his shoulders and looked directly at me. Then, without preface, conveyed the devastating information.

"Mrs. Duffy, as I suspected, you have Twin to Twin disease. There is a lot of fluid here. There is also a clear size difference—it appears that one of the babies has stopped growing." He scanned the instrument around my belly more fiercely, his eyes never leaving the screen.

I stared at the screen. I saw two little teddy grahams floating around the excess amniotic fluid. My heart thudded painfully, and my face felt hot. I closed my eyes to prevent the salty, fresh tears from streaming. I didn't know what the heck all of his words meant. My brain was on overload. The only information I could really process was the fact that one baby had stopped growing, and they were both in grave danger.

The pregnancy had started in a normal enough way. My husband Ed and I were both ecstatic that our family would be growing. The day after we found out we were having girls, we painted the spare bedroom a pale pink and purchased two matching cribs. Two years prior, we had been blessed as parents for the first time, and I'd been given the greatest title of all: mother to our daughter Abigail. But, though the positive pregnancy test made me feel like I was on cloud nine, my anticipatory excitement and happiness was tinged with fear. We'd suffered the traumatic and abrupt end to two previous pregnancies we thought had been healthy—one before Abigail and one after— and they had left us heartbroken. With our joy came unanswerable questions: What if something goes wrong? What if this pregnancy results in another miscarriage? What if the problem is me?

When I hit the seven weeks pregnant mark a couple of weeks later, the fear had finally started to dissipate. And then, abruptly, I started bleeding heavily, soaking through my clothes and onto the furniture. It was déjà vu; I'd done this all before. I thought I was having yet another miscarriage. Ed drove me to the ER and we waited what felt like hours to see a resident who of course couldn't tell us anything—until the Obstetrics attending arrived. When he arrived, he called for an emergency ultrasound. Since I was still so early in the pregnancy, I was subjected to the early ultrasound torture—the kind where the ultrasound wand—a long and narrow device—is inserted deep inside you. I laid back and placed my feet in the stirrups, and closed my eyes, dreading the words that were about to come out of this doctor's mouth. *Our baby is gone*, I thought to myself. Raising his eyebrows, the doctor turned to me.

"Wait a second, was this a spontaneous pregnancy?"

"Excuse me?" I wrinkled my forehead in confusion. What the heck was a spontaneous pregnancy? Was that like the Immaculate Conception?

"Err sorry, I mean, did you use fertility drugs?" he clarified.

"No. Why? We conceived our first child naturally—and fairly quickly might I add—we didn't need to."

"I see two heartbeats," he said and pointed to the screen. "Look, there's one flicker and there's the other." He turned from Ed, who stood silent and shocked, to me. "Right here is one amniotic sac, and up here, there's the other."

"Holy shit," Ed said as his expression changed to a smug smile. No doubt proud of what his super sperm had accomplished.

"Are you serious? Are you trying to tell me I have two babies in there?" I asked stupidly. Confusion and disbelief washed over me.

"Yes! You are having twins. Congratulations, Mr. and Mrs. Duffy!" he said as if he was awarding me a million bucks.

What I said next must have made me look and sound like a complete idiot.

"How is that possible?" Clearly my egg split somewhere along the way (or were there two eggs?). I tried to remember from biology class back in high school. Trying to recover from my stupidity, I quickly asked, "Are they identical or fraternal?"

"Too early for us to tell," he said continuing to study the ultrasound screen.

My feeling of shock was soon overcome by joy and excitement. Ed and I would be welcoming two little additions to our family.

"Ed, our prayers have been answered, God has given us two babies."

"I do see something else," he interrupted pausing to stare intently at the screen. *Oh gosh*, I thought. *Is there another baby in there?*

"There's your uterus, and the lining," he said mapping out my reproductive organs on the screen. "There's a blood clot in the uterus. That's the source of your bleeding and cramping." And there we had it.

"What does that mean, exactly?" I sat up on the table like a springboard, lowering my feet from the stirrups and pulling down the bottom of my gown. He sat down on his stool and scooted closer.

"We need to be very cautious," he said. "Sometimes these clots can pull the pregnancy and terminate it. In other cases, the clots will reabsorb themselves into your body and your pregnancy will continue as normal."

My brain was trying to catch up to my heart. I felt my joy swirl into fear. "Pull the pregnancy" and "terminate it." His words were blunt and graphic. This dangerous and potentially fatal condition was after my babies.

"Okay," I said pushing back a tear with my finger. "So what do we do?" I looked back at him for the answer. He got up from his stool and handed me a tissue.

"Mrs. Duffy, I suggest you follow up with your OB, but I would strongly recommend you stay on bed rest until the clot resolves." He grabbed his notepad from the counter and scribbled down the names of vitamins—ones I had never heard of. "You should double the dose of your prenatal vitamins and folic acid since there are two in there."

"Oh right, of course. That makes sense." I nodded in agreement.

I turned and looked back at the now blank ultrasound screen, and I thought: *There are two little babies in there, no bigger than a lentil, they have each other and are surrounded by amniotic fluid and a flipping blood clot.*

"All right Mrs. Duffy, you are all set," he said, putting his hand on my shoulder. "Remember to follow up with your doctor as soon as possible," he said, and walked out the door.

Pregnant with twins AND bed rest. That was a lot to digest all at once. Then, add to that a dangerous blood clot in my uterus that could make me lose them. I felt a sense of fury at this clot that had interjected itself into my healthy pregnancy. My own body was turning on me and trying to take away my babies. Well, I refused to succumb to this worst-case-scenario. I decided that losing this pregnancy and these babies was not an option.

Ed couldn't make it to the perinatologist appointment—he was taking a deposition. I wished he was sitting in the exam chair right beside me. Ed would know what to do. Ed would understand what was happening and what we needed to do to fix it. I had so many questions for Dr. Bill—the most important being: how are we going to save my babies? Nothing came out of my mouth except for anxious breathing.

After a few seconds, I calmed enough to ask Dr. Bill for clarification. I was hoping he might admit that he had made a mistake. He might take back his fateful words. He might say I was actually having a normal pregnancy and that my babies looked healthy. The room fell silent as I waited for his answer. I could hear Abby snacking on her Goldfish, but the iPad had been muted, and she stared at the screen silently. It seemed like this was happening to someone else in a parallel universe, not to me, like this was *Back to the Future*—Marty McFly's alternate version of 1985. Maybe if I walked outside there would be a DeLorean waiting to take me back to the real version of my life.

But it actually wasn't the first time I'd heard the term "Twin to Twin Disease." The possibility of this happening had been mentioned to me in the early doctor visits, but I'd discarded it because I had thought it would never apply to us. I thought it was just another example of the all-knowing and ever-hovering doctors laying out rare negative outcomes. I never imagined things would go wrong, this wrong. And then, in an instant, all the warnings I'd brushed aside came rushing back to me.

Dr. Cooper had told us when I was around twelve weeks pregnant that I was carrying Monochorionic-Diamniotic twins—Mono-Di.

"I see the membrane separating the two," he said studying the ultrasound screen.

"Oh okay, and what does that mean?"

"That tells us that your twins are in their own amniotic sac but share the same placenta."

The membrane is a big deal in twins. It's how they are able to distinguish the type of twins you are carrying. The sharing of the placenta—a monochorionic placenta—is a special characteristic of identical twins.

"Crystal, these types of twins can carry their own host of problems because they are at potential risk for twin to twin transfusion."

I didn't really understand what he meant by that, but I nodded because I wanted to move on and discuss other things I thought were more important and relevant. Just as with any pregnancy warning, I always thought: It's not going to be me, not *my* babies. No, that's the type of thing that only happens to 0.1 percent of people having twins, and they probably smoked and drank during their entire pregnancy. But I was wrong. Painfully wrong.

I sat there astounded as Dr. Bill unraveled more details of the horrific disease.

"Twin to twin transfusion syndrome—referred to as (TTTS) or Stuck Twin Syndrome—is a disease that affects the placenta, and it only occurs in identical twin pregnancies, because they share a placenta."

His delivery was nice enough, but this diagnosis still slapped me across the face. I should have been taking notes. But I couldn't move let alone write anything down. Didn't the doctor know how devastating this news was to me? I needed a moment to begin to wrap my mind around this and I needed some kind of hope before I dived into the dirty details.

But Dr. Bill was still talking. "The shared placenta contains abnormal blood vessels which connect the umbilical cord and the circulation of the twins."

"What in the world?" I heard all of the words he was saying, but I couldn't understand. I couldn't decipher the secret code. *What exactly is the problem*? I asked myself. The shock of the news was inhibiting me from processing information in any coherent way. He kept repeating "monochorionic placenta," "monochorionic-diamniotic," "donor," "recipient." I was getting lost in the medical jargon. I felt like Marty again, "English, Doc Brown." Then I immediately shifted into self-blame. Had I done something to cause this?

When I was five or six, I broke a Waterford crystal vase in our formal living room. My little sister Melissa was a toddler; we were playing tag and I was chasing after her. I ran into the side table knocking over the vase and spilling the hydrangeas that were arranged in it. There were shards of glass everywhere.

"It was all my fault," I burst into tears when I told my mom what had happened.

"That's okay, it was an accident," she reassured me. "You didn't do it on purpose."

I hadn't done it on purpose but I was old enough to know I should not have been running around in the formal living room—a room that millennials such as myself deemed unnecessary. I also knew how special that vase was to her, and well, I needed to assign blame to ease the guilt; it was no different with the TTTS diagnosis.

I feared I was somehow to blame. "So…" I cleared my throat. "How exactly did this happen?" "Did I do something to cause this?"

I was too active; I should have rested more. In fact, I never should have gone off bedrest. After the blood clot dissipated, I thought we were in the clear and nothing else could go wrong. I thought I could resume normal pregnant activities, including a family trip to Sea World. I had clearly pushed myself too far.

He shook his head. "No, it was nothing you did or didn't do. We aren't certain what causes TTTS. It is not genetic or caused by a specific thing. It just happens."

Why wasn't there an explanation? I wondered. Not even a medical theory based on facts? I did everything right. Why did this have to happen to us? I wanted answers no doctor could give me.

I felts the hot tears come and I stopped listening. I knew what this diagnosis meant: my twins were in the balance, hanging on for dear life. Voices were muddling, and then I heard Dr. Bill say something that caused me to stop breathing: "If not dealt with immediately, the mortality rate is 95 percent for both babies. In other words, there's a slim chance of survival."

"No." I gasped. I kept saying. "No, no, no, no, no." Hysteria gripped me.

"No, oh God, no!" my mom screamed, and my poor heartbroken dad put his face in his hands. Suddenly, I couldn't take any more. I sat up, and fiercely grabbed some tissues to wipe off the gunky gel from my stomach. I pulled my blouse down, stepped off of the exam chair and snatched my Tory Burch purse. I bent down and scooped up Abby into my arms. "Mommy, Mommy!" Abby kissed my cheek, a few Goldfish crumbs still on her little lips. *I'm outta here,* I thought. I hugged her and five seconds later walked out of the exam room.

CHAPTER 2

THE WAIT

The April sun glared hotly as I stormed out of the doctor's office into the parking lot. My mind felt like it had fractured into a million pieces. I could feel the surge of emotion coming. No, not yet, I thought. Just hold it together until I get home. But I felt the outpour would begin at any second—the hot, thick tears of fear, panic and utter horror. I was short of breath. I had to put Abby down next to me. I felt like I'd been punched in the chest and it had knocked the wind out of me. I continued to hold back the tears, suppressing them, waiting for the right moment to let go. It definitely wasn't here.

My parents caught up to me and Abby. My mom's face was splotchy, as if she'd been crying. She handed me a piece of paper with a name and number scribbled on it.

"The nurse stopped us on our way out," she said, using a tissue to wipe her nose. "They want you to go and see a specialist first thing in the morning, I'm…" her voice broke.

"I'm so sorry honey," she reached over and put her arms around me.

My dad reached into his pocket and handed me a small packet of tissues.

"A nurse from their office should be calling you," my dad said, now holding Abby by the hand.

I let go of my mom and took a step back. I opened my purse and pulled out my cell phone. My eyes widened as I looked at the screen.

"Seven missed calls," I screeched.

I had seven missed calls from Dr. Cooper, not the main office line, but his personal cell phone that he had given to me in case of an emergency. *Bad news travels fast.* I wondered if, at the moment I'd stormed out of the office, Dr. Bill had speed-dialed his colleague Dr. Cooper and relayed the upsetting news about his patient—the one he had referred to him months ago for additional screening. Dr. Cooper had been in the field for thirty years, he was confident with his decisions. After my second miscarriage, he had reassured me countless times, putting to bed my worries. He had a calm, cool and collected personality and spoke to me with such politeness and tact. His bedside manner was warm and soothing. Even when he didn't have the answers—especially the ones I wanted to hear—confiding in him had always made me feel better. He made me feel like a smart, well-researched and concerned mother-to-be rather than a paranoid pregzilla who was constantly on Web MD trying to self-diagnose. Things had been turned upside down, and my calm Dr. Cooper was now the one freaking out and calling me. *Yup,* I replied to Dr. Cooper in my head. *I'm aware that this-is-some-serious shit.*

The car ride home seemed longer than usual. I stared out of the window taking notice of the Houston Rodeo billboards. I looked forward to this time of year almost as much as I did Christmas. But eating barbeque and watching bull riders was the furthest thing on my mind. I picked up my cell phone, scrolled through my favorites list and dialed Ed's office line. I hated sharing awful news over the phone. He answered on the first ring and I blurted out, "We have Twin to Twin disease, the girls are sick."

"What?!" he cried in terror. I was sobbing into the phone, wiping my snot into my cheeks. I wasn't ready to repeat the details of the appointment. I told him we could talk about it more in person when he came home from work. I did not feel like talking and my parents definitely understood. No one wanted to talk. There was utter silence the entire twenty-five-minute car ride home.

As we pulled onto our street, I noticed another car in the driveway. It was parked in the spot right next to where I usually parked my minivan. It was Ed's gray Kia Forte. It was about 3:30 pm in the afternoon. Ed never left the office during the day unless it was for a deposition or client meeting. A habit instilled in him like most attorneys at big firms. Perhaps he had forgotten something at home that he needed? Perhaps he had spilled something at lunch and was coming home for a different shirt? Or a file for a really important case? Whatever the reason, I would soon find out. He stood there waiting for me in the driveway as we pulled in. He set his briefcase down against the door step and walked towards me. His ash brown hair with sprinkles of gray gelled neatly to the right side. He was wearing the navy-blue pinstripe suit that we had picked out together for his interview last fall with his current firm. It was perfectly fitted around his muscular, athletic build.

When I looked at him I noticed his sea-blue eyes were watery. In the decade I'd known him, I'd seen him cry twice—once at his great Aunt Kitty's funeral—she had passed away from lung cancer and he had been close with her growing up—and the second was after college when I'd threatened to break up with him once in the heat of an argument. I'd lost my temper and thrown my keys across the room in our apartment, and then, we spent the next couple of hours trying to find them. We didn't find them until the next morning as I hurried to get out the door for work—they were in a bookshelf behind a thick stack of law books. We laughed so hard we cried. We were such polar opposites, but while he may not be as obvious with his emotions to the entire world like I am, he feels just as much. There were no spoken words between us, only widened eyes that quickly filled up with tears. That was when I let it all go. Once those first few tears broke free, the rest followed in an unbroken stream. I sobbed convulsively into his chest— uncontrollably—having to remind myself to breathe. My dad picked up Abby and went inside along with my mom. I was thankful for that; no parent ever wants to break down in front of their child. This day, however, I gave myself a pass. This day, my fears and worst-case scenarios had unfolded right in front of me.

Ed put his hand on the back of my neck and massaged it slightly and whispered, "Crys, we'll get through this."

I wanted to believe him, but I wasn't so sure.

There was nothing that could be done now to undo the diagnosis, nothing except wait for the consultation the next morning.

Ed tucked me into our bed and lay with me for a few minutes, rubbing my back while I tried to fall asleep. He knew me so well. There were times I would talk his ear off over mindless nothings, and then there were times when my heart was aching and I just needed a quiet, loving and supportive partner. In his arms, and with his presence, at least I knew we would tackle this together. Just as we had in years past when we had lost our babies.

This would be possibly one of the worst night's sleeps of my life. Nothing helped me settle down—not fluffy pillows, down comforters or warm milk. I lay awake tossing and turning, replaying the day's events. Had I heard the doctor correctly? Maybe I misconstrued his words. Yes, that was it. That was clearly what had happened. *Ugh*, such baby brain. Double baby brain. I was unable to process all the information he'd thrown at me. In the morning, I'd realize it was all a misunderstanding, and I was still growing two healthy babies inside me. Unsurprisingly, the night was full of restless dreams. I fell asleep feeling the pain of that first miscarriage all over again.

We walked along the Hawaiian shore, hand in hand. We were twenty-six and it was the summer after our wedding. We giggled as the warm summer breeze sprayed a mist of saltwater on our faces. The water was sparkling blue; families were constructing sandcastles and gazing at the sea turtles napping mid-beach belly sunken into the sand. The catamarans were filled with tourists hoping to catch a glimpse of a whale. With each breath I took, I was mesmerized by the beauty of the coastline. Then, I turned and looked off into the distance and spotted a humpback whale about five-hundred feet back, breaching in midair as if to get our attention. And that she did.

"Wow, that is incredible, Ed—did you see that?" I exclaimed.

"Yeah, pretty cool, huh? That was always my favorite thing to do here as a kid, go on the whale watching tours…but funny, it's June, that's not typically whale season here." He raised his sunglasses to his forehead to get a better look.

"Oh really?" I said. "I kind of assumed they hung around here all year long."

"Nope, winter and spring you can see a ton of them. They travel in big pods." He paused and smiled sweetly. "You know, they come here all the way from Alaska to give birth to their calves, since it's warm and safe here from any predators."

"That is quite the hike for the pregnant mama whales." I paused and took a deep breath. "You know, I wouldn't mind giving birth here and then hanging out with the whales for a few months. We could become beach bums, get a place in Hana and have a little beach baby." I pulled down the bright pink polka dot rash guard that had started to rise up and expose my stomach.

"Ha, right!" he said shaking his head the way he usually did at my far-fetched ideas.

I turned back to sneer at him and stuck my tongue out playfully. He pulled his Ray Ban sunglasses back down over his eyes, and I could see bits of sunscreen on his freckled cheek that he hadn't rubbed in all the way.

"Hey, come here, you." I pulled him close to me and we plopped down on the beach, scattering sand all over us. I reached for his face and gently rubbed in the sunscreen. The mid-day sun was beating down with force. I reached into my beach bag, grabbed my tube of sunscreen and reapplied some more to his pale back.

"You know, you are going to be an amazing mother," he said, leaning in to kiss me. His radiant smile was a mile wide. "I can't wait. I'm going to be a daddy!" he said, reaching back over to me.

"I know, me too—I'm so excited—just eight months to go, little one!" I said rubbing my still completely flat tummy.

I'd spent the last six months or so leading up to this trip in full anticipation. I'd imagined the lush vegetation, expansive beaches and rolling white-capped waves. I was ready for sun, sand, surf and deep relaxation—time to tan on the beach and dream about our life together—and our new baby! What would he or she look like? Would she look like her daddy? Would he be a spitting image of me? Would she be sweet and smart like her father or extroverted and feisty like me?

We had the whole week mapped out—hiking in Hana to hidden waterfalls, surfing lessons on Kaannapali beach, snorkeling over coral reefs and sunset dinner cruises—toasting our happiness with grape juice. We took long walks on the beach, hand in hand, planning out the rest of our lives. This pregnancy had been a bit of an unexpected surprise, but we had wholeheartedly welcomed it. We both immediately fell in love with the thought of being parents. Even though we were young, we weren't overwhelmed or anxious by the change. This was our time—we had thought—to grow our family and grow in our love for one another.

We walked over to the little rental hut near our hotel—the one with all the brochures of life-changing adventures that the islands had to offer.

"Aloha, how can I help you?" asked the beautifully tanned and toned mid-twenties surfer working behind the bar.

"Aloha," Ed said proudly, as if he'd been to Hawaii a million times. That was almost true: Ed's family had visited every year, sometimes twice, since he was three. "We would like to rent some snorkel gear for the day."

"Of course, here are two masks and two pairs of fins," he said, handing Ed the gear. "They're yours for the day."

"Oh great!" I replied, thinking there was plenty of time for swimming, maybe even taking a nap on the beach and perhaps going back around sunset.

"Be sure to check out the reefs near Black Rock," said the surfer.

"Mahalo," I said as I grabbed my gear. I turned and look back at Ed; we were still standing in front of the equipment hut. "I can't believe I've never done this before. I can't wait to see schools of fish swimming around us."

"The reefs around Black Rock are incredible," Ed replied.

"How far of a swim is it?" I started to ask, but then a sudden, sharp pain in my abdomen stopped my words.

"Ouch!" I screamed.

Ed instinctively dropped the snorkel gear on the beach and put his arm behind my back. "Babe, what's wrong?"

"Ow!" I yelled again.

"Crystal, what's wrong!?" Ed said again.

"Really painful stomach cramps." I hunched over trying to breathe. "Just give me a sec," I said, trying to inhale and exhale deeply.

"Here, let's get you up to the room fast," Ed said as he scooped me up into his arms.

The scene back at our hotel room was a chaotic mess. I was hunched over on the couch screaming in pain. Ed sat beside me, frantically googling things on his laptop. He was repeating the words, "It's okay, don't worry, everything is going to be fine."

"I hope so," I choked out the words.

Heavy cramps were pounding inside me like an earthquake, burning like an inferno. I curled up in a ball on the foldout couch to ease the pain. I began to feel incredibly sick to my stomach. *Could this be morning sickness?* I thought to myself.

Then I felt it.

Blood started to trickle down slowly between my legs. I thought that was normal. Everyone said I might have some implantation bleeding. But it kept flowing and flowing. After several minutes, I knew something was definitely not right. I had already soaked through my board shorts and onto the palm tree printed pillow I'd been sitting in front of. I jumped up and dashed to the bathroom. I locked the door, still trying to convince myself everything was fine, and sat down, my toes curled up against the cold hard tile floor. With one hand on my stomach and the other gripping onto the wall, I let go and it all came flushing out. And then I looked down into the toilet bowl. I will never be able to get the horrifying image I saw there out of my head. I screamed in panic. I kept screaming until my throat was raw. Ed, who had been pounding on the door, demanding I let him in, finally kicked it open. He looked down and saw what I saw and gasped.

He reached for me and I collapsed into his arms.

When I opened my eyes, it was still dark outside; mist covered our bedroom windows. I sat up in the bed breathing deeply as I thought about the haunting memory of the painful nightmare I had already lived once. Each time the dream was a bit different; sometimes we would be snorkeling when it happened, other times we would be in the middle of a candlelight dinner on the beach. Each story ended in the same way. I lost our first baby in Hawaii that first summer after we were married, and then two years later, lost our second baby on a trip to Las Vegas. The memory of losing our two babies still haunted me and the fear was now projecting itself onto our twin pregnancy.

How I wished the Twin to Twin diagnosis had been just a nightmare. Nightmares ended when you woke up, and everything returned to normal. I turned to look at Ed, who had fallen asleep with a laptop on our comforter. He'd been awake most of the night researching TTTS, carrying the panic and fear for both of us.

I nudged his arm gently.

"Did that really happen?" I softly whisper. "Wait. Before you answer, just tell me it didn't. Tell me I dreamt it."

He sighed. He couldn't tell me what I so badly wanted to hear.

"Are we actually going to talk to a specialist today about some bizarre blood transfusion disease?" I asked.

"I'm afraid so," he replied groggily.

"I'm scared," I confessed.

"Me too," he said as he hugged me tightly. He held me in bed for a long time. As we got dressed, he went over some of his findings of TTTS with me, the parts he left out were too terrifying for me to even imagine. I had decided that, in a desperate attempt to avoid complete distress, I was going to stay off the internet. I did not want to terrorize myself with unknowns or potential scenarios of TTTS. In order to survive this, to beat this, the babies—our girls—needed to be calm and soothed, which meant I needed to be that way as well. If I was a nervous wreck, they would feel that and feed off of it. It was far easier to hear what I needed to know about this disease from Ed. It was hard to keep all the details straight, but I wanted to walk into the Maternal-Fetal Medicine (MFM) office and feel a little familiar with some of the terms they would use.

Ed explained to me what Dr. Bill had tried to the day before—that because our girls were identical and shared a placenta, they had many abnormal blood vessels that connected their umbilical cords and circulatory systems. Depending on a number of factors— blood type and direction of the flow—blood could be transfused disproportionately from one twin (known as the donor) to the other twin (known as the recipient). The transfusion caused the donor twin to have decreased blood volume, and in turn, a slower growth than the co-twin. If the donor twin had poor urinary output, that could cause low amniotic fluid—another big potential problem. The recipient baby, on the other hand, could become overloaded with blood. This superfluous amount of blood would strain this baby's heart to the point that it might actually develop heart failure. I took a deep breath. I knew we had a long day ahead of us.

CHAPTER 3

THE LONGEST DAY

Even though the perinatologist's office was in the same
building as Dr. Cooper's office, it felt somehow like we were in another
world completely. A world where pregnancies had gone awry. We had
been sent to the Texas Fetal Center, which was across the sky bridge
close to the children's hospital. The center specialized in fetal care for
babies with congenital anomalies or genetic abnormalities. During
my pregnancy with Abby, I had read all about these centers and all
the details of genetic testing for abnormalities and fetal interventions.
I knew how lucky we had been both then and now. I had always felt
blessed that my pregnancy with her had been uneventful.

We were meeting with an MFM Specialist, who was an expert in
diagnosing and treating high-risk pregnancy complications including
TTTS. Ed held my hand as we walked into the office; my nerves were
completely shot. I was freezing, but my palms were oddly sweaty. I
felt nauseated, and a lump started to form in the back of my throat.
Breathe, I just needed to focus on breathing. I squeezed Ed's hand
so tight that his wedding ring dug into my finger. The reception area
looked more like the inside of a home—a parlor sofa against the wall
and an arm chair to the side. There was a frosted glass window; Ed
tapped on the glass. The window slid open and we were greeted by a
petite, blonde nurse. She was young, about twenty-three or twenty-four.
She wore thick, black-rimmed glasses, had her hair pulled back in a
ponytail and wore light blue scrubs with little black and white Snoopys
all over. Charles Schultz's Snoopy reminded me of Abby. When she
was a newborn, during middle of the night feedings, I always had the TV
on to help me stay awake. I often watched old reruns of *Peanuts* since
it was the only thing on. One of Abby's first stuffed animals had been a

tiny Snoopy that sang the theme song when you pressed its stomach. She took that Snoopy everywhere with her. My warm memories of Abby deflected my nerves and calmed me.

"Hi Mr. and Mrs. Duffy, she said. "we have been expecting you. I'm Jessica, the nurse coordinator—we spoke last night on the phone." She reminded me as if there was any chance I had forgotten. I nodded in acknowledgment. "If you will follow me, please," she said and signaled for us to enter the hallway.

For the first time in my pregnancy history, I had no wait time. Efficiency at a doctor's office was never a good sign. I saw it as underscoring the severity of my condition. We were immediately escorted from the comfortable waiting area and into one of the exam rooms. Jessica pulled out a chair from against the wall so I could sit. She opened up a green binder, which I could only assume was our chart, and scanned the documents. She started a long list of questions. She carefully noted everything we said, smiled and looked up at us.

"I think I have everything I need for now. Our sonographer will be in shortly to do your ultrasound."

I leaned back in my chair, trying to find a comfortable position—an impossible task when you have a bowling ball under your blouse. There was zero chance of this experience being anything but unpleasant and unsettling.

There was a knock on the door about two minutes later. A young brunette, probably about my age, came in holding our chart.

"I'm going to be doing your ultrasound today," she said. "If you can sit on the exam chair, we can go ahead and get started."

I slid off the waiting room chair and hoisted myself on the exam chair. I lie back slowly. I felt like a snail gliding along the leather; if only I could bury and retract into my shell to avoid predators the way they do.

"You okay, sweetie?" Ed said offering me his arm.

"Not really," my voice was soft and low. "But I just want to get this over with."

He nodded in agreement.

I opened my mouth and began to say, "I think once—" but the tech cut me off midsentence.

"I need you to stop talking please, so I can concentrate on the ultrasound. I need it to be quiet."

She lacked bedside manner—to say the least. Come on, chick, I wanted to tell her. *I know this is your job and you see "cases" like me all the time, but would it kill you to smile and be nice? We are going through a lot right now.*

My ultrasound scans with Dr. Cooper were always quick, lasting only about five minutes, and with Dr. Bill in the past couple of months, they had usually lasted around twenty minutes. But today with tech Barbie, it felt like the scan took forever. I looked up at the clock on the wall and saw an entire hour had gone by. *How much longer?* Ed and I sat in complete silence as she continued to scan my belly. *Scan, glide across, repeat. Scan, glide across, repeat.* She said nothing, only grimaced, and meticulously jotted her findings in a notebook.

A few times I interrupted the silence and asked, "What do you see?" or "What does that mean?" Her reply was always delivered in a stoic tone.

"The doctor is really the best one to go over the ultrasound findings with you. I'm not supposed to say anything."

"Well can I ask, sorry, how much longer is this going to be?" I lowered my head expecting her to bite it off.

"We can take a break if you need to sit up, but it will just delay us."

"When you are twenty-three weeks pregnant with twins, its painful to be in any position for a long time, let alone on my back," I said, rolling my eyes.

"Let me just finish measuring the amniotic fluid, and then I can send in the heart sonographer to meet with you."

Heart sonographer? Oh right, to look at the babies' hearts—another thing Ed had read about online.

"Okay," I said. Ed and I exchanged glances, like prisoners in custody awaiting our fate. We resumed sitting in nervous silence and awkwardness until she finished. As I waited, I couldn't help but think about the other patients there. Was there another mom going through this on the other side of the wall? Another mom and dad scared for the health and safety of their baby's life? How many tears were shed in this office daily?

When the tech Barbie left the room, the heart sonographer walked in as if on cue. He was a young guy in his mid-thirties with red-hair and freckles. I wanted to break the ice and say something—a heart joke—anything to try and lighten the intensity in the room.

"Hearts will never be made practical until they can be made unbreakable," I said smiling gently.

"Excuse me?" he looked at me in utter confusion.

"It's from *The Wizard of Oz*?" Ed said.

"Yes," I nodded. "One of our favorites—we watch it with our little girl."

"Oh okay," the tech said.

He didn't introduce himself, he just told me that we needed to get started with the exam.

It seemed odd to allow a stranger to massage oil all over my belly—what is normally a very intimate act. Even more than that, I permitted a stranger to peer into the world of my womb to determine what had gone awry before Ed and I knew. And, all the while, we exchanged so few words. Shouldn't Ed and I be the first to know? Shouldn't the techs be giving us a play-by-play of the action? We wanted to know what he could see and gather from the ultrasound.

Specifically, what damage had the blood transfusion caused? Were the babies' hearts okay? And their bladders? Would we have to have surgery? Would this cause the babies any lasting effects?

Ed tried asking again, but the tech just smiled and said it was best to wait for Dr. Miller to explain everything fully. We continued with the scans and endured more egregious waiting for them to be completed. When he was done with his analysis, he left the room. We waited some more. In total, we waited about two hours. The pressure was building in my back, and my sciatic nerve hurt like hell. How much more of this torture would I have to withstand? Finally, Jessica came back into the room.

"Dr. Miller will discuss the results with you now," she said extending her arm to help me out of the exam chair. "Come right this way to the conference room."

We were finally going to find out the severity of the disease. Terror manifested itself. deep inside me. I could feel the chunks of bagel I'd had for breakfast threatening to forcefully come back up. I took a deep breath and wiped my sweating palms on my skirt. The consultation room was very different from the waiting area. It was what I imagined a modern-day psychiatric hospital room would look like. The walls were blank—no posters of sleeping newborns, no floral artwork, no seaside landscapes, no TV—nothing but white-painted sheetrock and laminate floors. There was a tiny window on the far-right wall, and in the middle of the room stood a round, wooden table with cushioned chairs. There was a large whiteboard on the opposite wall and a side table stocked with different colored Expo markers and erasers. Jessica turned and left the room, and a brief few seconds later, a tall doctor appeared in the doorway. He was wearing dark blue scrubs and looked as if he just came out of surgery. He pulled off his hat and introduced himself.

"Hello there, Mr. and Mrs. Duffy, I'm Dr. Andrew Miller. Call me Andy. I'm one of the MFMs here at the Fetal Center." He had a gentle voice— not soft, but not abrasive either. He had piercing blue eyes and a moustache; his hair was gray with traces of white. He reached for our file which Jessica had set on the table.

"Why don't we all have a seat," he motioned for us to sit around the conference table. "Can we get you two anything to drink? Or a snack?"

"Oh yes please, I'll take a water and anything you have to munch on." I said rubbing my grumbling belly.

"I'll grab you a water and a chocolate chip cookie," Jessica said leaping up from her chair. "And I'll grab one for Dad too."

"Thanks Jess," Dr. Miller said, and then turned his attention back to us.

"So I've just looked over the results of the ultrasound scans we did here today." He paused.

This is it. How bad can it be? Not that bad—right? Or tragically, irreversibly bad? My thoughts ricocheted from best-case to worst-case and back again.

"Before we begin, I just want to give you a little background about myself. I'm one of the few MFMs in the country that specializes in twin to twin transfusion cases. I'm one of the pioneers who trained in Europe when these surgeries were being developed. I also teach at the medical school here and have published a ton of articles on Twin to Twin cases that I've seen over the years. I want you to rest assured that you are in the best of hands with us."

A high-risk pregnancy genius with a passion for TTTS. He sounded heaven-sent.

He opened our chart, did one last skim and then closed it shut again.

"Guys," his blue eyes widened as he looked both me and Ed in the eye.

"Let me give you an analogy," he said.

"Imagine a tornado has just formed up north in Oklahoma. It's formed out of nowhere, faster than any meteorologist could have predicted. Now, this tornado may destroy everything in its path, or it may dissolve, leaving only slight winds and light rain with minor damage. That's similar to how TTTS works."

"Oh, my goodness!" I interrupted, "What do you mean?"

"Well, I've just spent the morning looking at your chart, reviewing your history and past reports from Dr. Bill's notes. It appeared as though everything in your pregnancy was going as it should have. Look here," he opened to a page in our file and pointed at the top, "it shows on this timeline that you were going to Dr. Bill every two weeks as a precaution per your OB's request." He paused. "Every two weeks is great, it's exactly what we recommend high-risk pregnant moms to do."

"Okay, good," Ed said, nodding in agreement. I said to myself, So, we were doing what we were supposed to be doing and… your point?

"You went to Dr. Bill the second week of April. There was no excess amniotic fluid showing at that time, and you hadn't experienced any symptoms."

He lowered his finger and pointed to another date. "Here, you returned to see Dr. Bill at your usual two-week mark, and discovered that not only are your babies suffering from TTTS, but it has already progressed to stage three within a matter of days."

"Oh no!" I gasped. "Like a tornado, out of anyone's radar." I screwed my eyes shut and put my head into my hands.

"The best case scenarios are when we can diagnose TTTS very early on in the pregnancy at around weeks fifteen to eighteen, at which point we just monitor the mom and babies and see how the TTTS progresses. Sometimes, the only thing necessary is to drain some of the excess amniotic fluid—nothing invasive—but in your case, it has developed further along in the pregnancy, so there are different courses of action." And then he backed up and explained.

"My point with the tornado analogy is not to scare you, but I want you guys to know that this disease is crazy and unpredictable, like a tornado. There's things we can do to monitor and correct problems, but we can never be absolutely positive of the outcome. We can only hope for the best."

"So, Dr. Miller, how bad is it?" Ed asked.

Dr. Miller minced no words.

"Looking at the results of the scans, it's apparent that one of the twins—Baby A—is very sick."

"Oh no, Baby A! That's Katherine—our little Katie," I shrieked.

"How? What specifically?" Ed interrupted.

"Well, you see, the transfusion that has occurred here between the twins has resulted in Baby B, who we call the donor twin, to experience low blood volume. So, our focus with this baby is that she is growing at a slower rate than her sister."

"That's Lauren—Baby B—is Lauren Elizabeth," I said. I wanted to identify these babies that he was analyzing from charts as real live individuals. They were our daughters. The medical terms were starting to annoy me. They were so impersonal.

"And with the recipient twin—err Katie," he corrected himself, "her heart has been overloaded with blood from her sister. All this excess blood has put a strain on her heart and…" He paused for a moment.

"She's in heart failure right now. If we don't operate, there's a 90 percent chance that both babies will die."

He stopped talking. I stopped breathing. What? Die? Are you kidding me?

I started silently panicking. I couldn't wrap my mind around the doctor's words. My stomach was cramping. I tried hunching over which made the pain in my back from lying on it during the scans worse. I wanted to scream. I wanted to throw something—perhaps the chair I was sitting on—across the room. And then throw up—that was how nauseated I was. I could feel my face turning burning red as I choked back tears. I couldn't look in Dr. Miller's direction any more. I turned away—I wanted to turn my thoughts to something else.

We had just received the results of the blood screening. It was time to reveal the gender of the babies.

"GIRLS! TWO MORE GIRLS, NO WAY!" I screamed when Dr. Cooper told me.

My heart skipped a beat. I was still beaming at the news that we were having identical twins, and finding out that they were girls sent me over-the-moon. It was absolutely precious. Three little girls. Half a pep squad, ha-ha. Maybe they would all have Abby's sparkling blue eyes? But really, I was just happy that we were having two healthy babies. I couldn't have cared less about the gender.

Then I turned to look at Ed—my best friend and life partner. Over the years, I'd told him countless times, "I couldn't do this life with anyone else but you." We completed each other so well. I was the CEO of the Duffy household—in charge of all day-to-day operations—and he was the Chairman of the Board—in charge of finances, and together, we made large decisions. Would he be okay not having a son? Not having that little boy to bond with, play catch with or take to Cubs games.

I turned towards him and leaned in closer.

"So, it looks like you and Charlie, our pup, are desperately outnumbered," I said jokingly.

And then I said, "But seriously, are you okay with us not having a son?"

He leaned in and kissed my forehead. "Why do I need a boy? Abby encompasses anything I could have ever imagined my child to be—she adores me and shares so many of my interests—soccer, *Star Wars*, Cinnamon Toast Crunch… Girls can do anything boys can do, and honestly, I'm honored that I get to raise her and instill that confidence and belief in her and our other daughters."

I fell in love with him all over again.

We came up with the girls' names together, well half of them anyway. We had both always loved Katherine for its traditional and royal sound, and we would call her Katie for short. It was derived from the Greek word *Hekateros*, which means "each of the two." Fitting for a twin. Her middle name would be Maria, after my mom. For Baby B, we thought long and hard as to what would go with Katherine. We loved the names Olivia, Emily, and Michelle—my middle name, and a family name from my side. But ultimately, while chatting with my aunt Michelle one day, who was pregnant with her third little boy, she confided in me that, if she had had a girl, she would have named her Lauren Elizabeth. I fell in love with the name immediately. And then just like Rachel took Monica's baby girl name on Friends, I took Michelle's. I asked her if it was okay, to which she replied, "Of course." With that, it was settled. Our twin girls would be Katherine Maria and Lauren Elizabeth.

That happy day seemed so far away. I blinked and shook my head, trying to regain focus, and saw that Dr. Miller had leaned in closer to Ed.

"A year ago, I would have done this procedure immediately. But they've been doing some experimenting with a drug called Nifedipine to bolster the recipient baby's heart. Taking this medication for twenty-four hours before the surgery will increase Baby A's chances of survival."

My head was still spinning. I only heard half the words he spoke. I was doing everything in my power to try to keep it together. I didn't want to toss furniture, and I didn't want to break down and cry in the room either. At the least, sobbing would have distracted me from getting all the necessary information. While I knew I could count on Ed—who was frantically taking notes and no doubt would remember every detail—I wanted to listen closely for myself to make the best possible decision for my girls. I couldn't mess this up. I had to be strong for my girls. This thought calmed me and infused me with a tinge of courage.

"Okay, so you think the best course of action is to get Crystal started on this heart medication and then do the surgery the next day?" asked Ed.

"Yes," Dr. Miller said, nodding. "I do, I think it is our best shot at beating this thing."

"What exactly does the surgery entail?" Ed asked.

"We will put Crystal completely under and basically take a laser in utero and cut all the blood vessels connecting the girls to each other. This will separate the placentas so that each baby is in her own placental sac. Right now, they are sharing a placenta, which—as you guys know—is what caused this problem.

Wait a sec, Jedi master, I thought. *What is this,* The Empire Strikes Back? *You want to laser inside me? That's insane. The girls were created from one egg splitting. They were intended to share a placenta. Won't trying to create two placentas harm the girls?*

But I was unable to vocalize my concerns. As he continued to describe the surgery, I kept imagining my girls—so vulnerable, being operated on before they even entered the world. *What a way to start a life.* Ed and Dr. Miller proceeded to discuss the details of the surgery. It was all getting too intense. I wanted to wipe the sweat off my face and blow my nose. I quickly scanned the room and spotted one lone box of tissues on the side table next to the whiteboard with all the Expo markers. There was no point in trying to reach for it because it was so far. Who put only one damned box of tissues in the conference room of doom where a stream of bad news had been given to other parents in our situation? I could have tried to signal Ed to pass it to me, but he was in the middle of a serious discussion with Dr. Miller, and I didn't want to interrupt.

Dr. Miller made eye contact with me. It felt like a college professor had just caught me talking to a friend instead of paying attention during a lecture.

"We will also drain the excess fluid which has made you feel bloated. This may make you feel lighter and more comfortable," he paused and smiled gently.

"We also need to talk about our plan if it looks like one baby isn't going to make it," he said. "If one baby dies, usually the other will too… unless we intervene. So, we have the option of tying off the umbilical cord of the dying baby to try and save the other, a process called umbilical cord occlusion."

Holy shit! How had things come to *this*? I couldn't take it anymore. I sprang up from my chair and made a beeline to the bathroom. As I sprinted out the door, I heard his voice trail off.

"I'm so sorry, I know this is incredibly difficult. I'll give you and Crystal a few minutes to process this information."

I stood in front of the bathroom mirror with tears streaming down my cheeks. *This is a choice I can't make. Selective termination? How could we ever choose to save one baby over the other?*

It reminded me of *Sophie's Choice,* the William Styron novel I'd read years earlier in college. It was during World War II, Sophie, the protagonist, had just arrived at Auschwitz concentration camp with her ten-year-old son and seven-year-old daughter when a sadistic Nazi told her that she could only bring one of her children. One would be killed so the other could live. She was forced to choose, and now Ed and I were being forced to choose. Or at least be open to that option.

I'm not doing this. There is no way! I told my reflection. *We are not having this conversation.*

I turned on the faucet and splashed cold water on my face and neck. I mopped off my face with a paper towel, took a deep breath and left the bathroom. I opened the door of the conference room of doom. Dr. Miller wasn't there, and Ed rushed over to me.

"You okay?" He placed his hand on my back.

"No! I just can't," I screamed.

"How can we just give up on one of our babies?" My eyes filled with tears. "How could we live with ourselves, Ed?"

"Yes, but how could we live with ourselves if both babies died and we could've saved one?"

I already knew what it was like to lose an unborn child—and I couldn't bear the thought of it happening again.

"Well, let's just hope it never comes to that," I said. "I have my answer."

The door creaked open and Dr. Miller walked back in.

"I'm so sorry, guys. I know how scary this is. Hell, I try to put myself in your position and think about what I would do." He smiled. "I'm used to delivering this kind of news to couples on a daily basis, and it never gets easier. Anything I can answer or go over with you? You can take the evening and think about this decision you have to make. I'll follow up with you first thing in the morning when you check-in for pre-op."

Neither one of us spoke a word. Ed shook his head, indicating we understood.

"Crystal, don't forget to pick up your prescription," he said, tearing off the small sheet with his scribbled signature and handing it to me.

"The sooner you get started on that, the better chance of survival for baby Katie. Try to get some rest, both of you. We have a long day ahead of us tomorrow. We will do everything we can, and then it's in God's hands."

LASER ABLATION

Two small red pills. Nifedipine was a channel blocker
designed to relax the muscles of my heart and blood vessels in order
to give baby Katherine a fighting chance. I poured the pills from the
prescription bottle into my hand and just stared at them. These two
tablets—each no bigger than a watermelon seed—held the fate of
my baby. Would they work? Would they do what they were designed to
do? Would they relax her little heart, which had been pumping overtime
because of the blood transfusion exchange between her and her
sister? I held them in my hand, closed my eyes and prayed. Please
work. Please help my baby. Please help baby Katherine. Please
flipping work.

I had another sleepless night. I was mildly dizzy and had a
headache—a common side effect from the drugs. I tossed and turned,
checked the clock, attempted to calm myself, tried different positions,
got up and paced and started the process all over again. The few
times I dozed off, my subconscious worries morphed into frightening
scenarios of the next day's events. In one dream, I watched as my
babies were swept out to sea in a cradle. I swam as hard as I could, but
I couldn't reach them in time. When they disappeared, I dove down into
the depths of the ocean to save them, but I couldn't hold my breath long
enough and nearly drowned. I awoke gasping for breath.

Without a doubt this laser ablation surgery would be a life-altering
procedure Would our doctors be able to save both our babies from this
dangerous disease? If the dreaded scenario occurred, would they be
able to save at least one baby?

I had had so many tearful moments since our diagnosis—tears of terror, anger and confusion. But I was beginning to move past that. I realized my worrying wasn't going to change the problems we faced. And, most importantly, I truly believed that the twins and I were one entity. Whatever I felt, they felt, whether it was joy or sadness and everything in between. If I let myself surrender to darkness, depression and negative thoughts, I feared my outcome would be darkened as well. I had to change. I had to no longer allow myself tears of terror, anger and sadness—no more worries or anxiety, only faith. Positive thoughts of hope and lots of prayers. It took everything in me to overshadow this frightening place and remember the happy moments of my life.

I relived my first moments alone with Abby. It was several hours after she was born. The hospital had gotten quiet: My visitors one by one had trickled out, the doctors were gone, the night nurses were at their stations, and Ed was fast asleep on the couch. My room was dark—only a small light in the side room was turned on. It was just me and Abby. The nurse had placed her in a clear plastic bassinet beside my bed. She was all swaddled up like a burrito—the pink, crochet baby blanket my mom had made was draped over her. She wore a pink and blue striped hospital cap with a little bow strung through the top that my nurse had made. I leaned over the rail on my hospital bed and carefully picked her up.

I held her in my arms which rested on my sore, deflated stomach. She was sleeping. I held her close to my face and breathed her in. Her fresh, sweet and immensely satisfying scent enthralled me. She smelled so delightful—like nothing I'd ever before experienced in my life. Somehow, her smell triggered a euphoric high in me. I sat there cradling her, gently rocking her back and forth and then she wiggled: her feet kicked—just as they had countless times when I was pregnant—as if trying to break free. She opened her eyes, her big beautiful blue eyes, and looked right at me. I gazed into her eyes, completely mesmerized by her power over me. It was in that moment, when it was just the two of us, that I looked at her and knew that there would never be a greater joy. I was holding my baby, this new life that Ed and I had created. She was finally here—this new person that would forever be connected to me. The elation that came from giving life to another human being would be unmatched by any other life experience. I knew for certain that I was meant to do it again someday, and this time I'd be bringing two lives into the world simultaneously. I lay in my bed, envisioned the happy outcome and felt it with my entire being.

I prayed nonstop that night before my surgery:

Lord, please help us and see us through this surgery. I ask that you be with the doctors and the surgeons tomorrow—that your steady hand be on theirs, guiding them as they do what they must do to safeguard the precious lives of my baby girls. Please, please, please.

We arrived at the hospital around 6:00 a.m. for our pre-op meeting with Dr. Miller.

"Right this way, Mrs. Duffy," said the pre-op nurse. "If you'll get undressed, and remove any jewelry or make-up then put on this gown. The doctor will be here shortly."

A few minutes later, Dr. Miller—our high risk-pregnancy genius, in whom I had great confidence—entered the pre-op room, accompanied by a nurse wheeling a sonogram machine. The nervousness I had suppressed over the previous thirty-six hours rushed over me. I recalled Dr. Miller's words: "A year ago, I would have done the surgery immediately. But we've found that waiting a day after administering this medication will increase the chances that the recipient baby survives the surgery."

I let myself fully realize what that meant: the danger my babies faced was not only real, but imminent, and with each passing moment, things could get worse. As I thought about the dire situation, I could not help but fear that the darn little red pills had failed to do their job. That my little recipient baby, Katie, could already be gone. The dread only grew when the nurse turned on the machine, and Dr. Miller began moving the sensor around. I felt conflicted—I wanted to know the truth, but I didn't really. If Katie was already gone, I would be devastated. I didn't know how I would be able to get through this surgery already knowing the outcome. Ed was right beside me, throughout the entire scan, holding my hand and reminding me to just breathe deeply. *Just get through the next couple of minutes.*

Peering at the screen, I could make out two shadowy shapes. The sonogram picture bounced around and shifted shape whenever the nurse touched it, making it impossible to discern anything, much less know if it was good or bad. I knew they were my babies, but like the day before, I couldn't tell what was going on or whether the scene on the monitor was good, bad or inconclusive. I knew Dr. Miller knew, and as he opened his mouth to speak, I braced for the worst.

To my relief, he said, "It looks like we still have both babies." It wasn't exactly a ringing endorsement; the status quo had been preserved, but the status quo wasn't exactly optimistic. Then Dr. Miller's slight smile conveyed that the twins' condition might actually be looking up.

"Look here," he said to us as he pointed to the screen, "you can see that the ventricles in the recipient's heart are showing improved diastolic flow." The nurse smiled and nodded.

Although I couldn't completely understand the medical jargon, I knew that hearing "improve" and "heart" in the same sentence was a good thing.

Dr. Miller continued, "It's quite remarkable to see this level of improvement after just twenty-four hours of the Nifedipine treatment."

Thank you, little red pills. Ed grabbed my hand and squeezed. *Finally,* I thought. *Maybe we turned a corner.* Things were starting to improve—my calmness and positive energy had paid off. But we were by no means out of the woods yet. Hell, we hadn't even had the laser ablation surgery yet, nor did we know whether it would even be feasible. But, for the first time since Dr. Bill had given us the dreaded diagnosis, we had a piece of good news. My babies were both alive, and they were already starting to feel better.

After hearing the news, I felt a bit more relaxed—maybe a bit too relaxed. A different nurse came in to start my IV and give me blood pressure-reducing medication—standard operating procedure before the surgery. Thankfully, Ed noted that I had already had a dose of Nifedipine, the same blood pressure-reducing medication the nurse wanted to give me, earlier that morning as one of Dr. Miller's instructions to increase the chance that the recipient twin survived the surgery.

"Oh, thanks," the nurse said nonchalantly. "It definitely wouldn't be good for you to take a second one, especially since your blood pressure is low already; the last thing we need is for you to have heart problems from an overdose."

I rolled my eyes in my husband's direction and thought, *Good thing you were paying attention, Ed.*

A few more minutes of waiting and I was ready to be rolled down to the OR. Dr. Miller came into the room again, this time accompanied by Dr. Cooper who wanted to check on me before the procedure.

Dr. Miller asked us whether we had decided what to do if they determined they could only save one of the babies. Ed and I had discussed this the night before. The ethical and practical dilemmas posed by this question were immense. Dr. Miller had explained that, if one of the twins had already died in utero or was in a chronic condition, the other twin would almost surely follow unless drastic steps were taken. Basically, the surviving twin would panic and die if she realized her sister was gone. The only way to stop this from happening was to block the supply of blood and nutrients to the twin that had passed (or would soon pass).

In the little time we had the night before, Ed had consulted our priest, Fr. Matthews, who had met with us several times before we were married as part of our Catholic wedding preparations. The twin to twin diagnosis was terrifying. And I wondered how I could be the one to decide the fate of one of my babies, knowing that it might lead to the death of both babies. Catholic doctrine is not perfectly clear on the subject. Generally, Catholicism opposes any intentional action on an unborn baby that would kill it (even in the case of ectopic pregnancies). But how did those teachings, or any ethical rules, apply in a situation where neither would survive if "nature ran its course" while killing one might save the other? How could someone weigh the survival of one's child against the moral opprobrium of killing one's other child? It was the worst paradox that a parent could imagine.

Even though there was a slim chance it would come to this, it was a horrifying dilemma. I understood that for some families this may be their best option, which is why Dr. Miller presented it. But for us, we decided that Dr. Miller and his team should try to save both, even if this reduced the likelihood of the healthier twin surviving. But, we said, if there was no chance of Katie surviving, we authorized them to do whatever they needed to save Lauren. Either way it was a nightmare, and I prayed it wouldn't come to that. These unthinkable Sophie's Choice scenarios weren't what I wanted to discuss before the operation, so I cleared my mind of the possibilities and returned my focus to the positive news we'd heard: both girls were alive and doing better.

Another thought came to mind. They were taking me to the same operating room where I delivered Abby two years earlier. Dr. Cooper scheduled a C-section when Abby was breech and I started having contractions. I was awash with very different emotions this time around. Because Abby was my first baby, everything had been new and I balanced a mix of feelings—mainly excitement, but a tad bit of nervousness too. Throughout my pregnancy with her, I had felt calm, safe and reassured. Of course, I had my worries, as with any pregnancy, but I mainly focused on my pregnancy winnings. I had managed to escape prolonged nausea, stretch marks and hemorrhoids. I was slightly worried about Abby's size in relation to my petite frame and how we would get her out safely. It was something we had talked about since the very beginning. I recalled those early appointments with Dr. Cooper in which Abby was measuring unusually big.

"I'm not sure your body is going to be able to labor naturally with this girl, kiddo," Dr. Cooper said.

I had the vision of doing everything naturally—I had contemplated a home birth to re-enact what my grandmother Ita did seven times—but it wasn't in the cards for me. I was thankful to have been born in a time of medical advances which saved my and my baby's life. Abby had been in downward position almost the entire time and then decided to flip in my third trimester. I knew trying to get babies to flip back around could be a tricky proposition, so when I woke up that stifling hot July morning with labor pains, I knew we needed to take the quick, safe route and have the C-section. Turns out I made the best decision for us.

"We made the right call, kiddo," Dr. Cooper told me later. "You could have labored for two days and then we still would have had to do an emergency C-section."

Even with the urgent C-section, I knew that my baby would be robust, that I'd be able to hold her right away and that she'd be going home with us within a few days.

This pregnancy was the polar opposite. It had been a struggle from day one and hadn't let up since. Every day brought new challenges. I had no idea what to expect. The positive readings earlier that morning gave me hope that the fear and difficulties had crested, but I knew that wasn't the case. It felt strange to be wheeled to OR #2 where my pregnancy with Abby had ended. Definitively. Safely. Positively. Joyfully. This time around it wasn't the final destination, but merely one stop along a very long and uncertain road.

Another difference: when they had delivered Abby, I was fully conscious; they just used a local anesthetic. This time, I'd be knocked out and completely unaware of my unfurling fate. Will the surgery have worked? Will they have had to sacrifice one baby for another? Or will they have saved both baby girls? I agonized over the decision Ed and I had made, but tried to stay focused on the little bit of good news we'd received and remembered the incredibly positive outcome the last time I had been in this operating room. I wanted to believe that magic was present, as it had been two years earlier. I remembered Abby's first cries—her grand entrance into the world—and our first days with her in the hospital. My last thought before the anesthesia set in was, *Things are in God's hands and in the hands of Dr. Miller and his team.*

CHAPTER 5

WHAT DO WE DO NOW?

I slowly emerged from an anesthesia-induced slumber to the incessant beeping of the heart and oxygen monitors. There was a dull pressure from the IV in my arm. The elastic, adhesive tape had been wrapped around tight and was digging into my skin. And of course, there was the nausea that never seemed to fully dissipate. Ed was at my bedside, holding my hand. He asked me how I was doing.

"To be honest, I feel much less like a blowfish," I croaked, my throat a bit raw from the anesthesia.

Ed laughed. "You look less like one."

I would've slapped him if I didn't have an IV stuck in my arm.

He told me that the surgery had gone really well. Dr. Miller said both girls looked okay; he had been able to get a good separation of the placenta, meaning that the fluid imbalance and the blood flow problems should improve. After the laser ablation was done and the blood vessels had been blocked, which apparently only took fifteen minutes, Dr. Miller drained the excess fluid from the recipient's side of the sac. This apparently relieved a lot of the pressure that I had been feeling—the reason I knew something was wrong in the first place.

"But, Houston, we do have another problem," Ed said.

"Are you serious? What now?"

"So, the doc nicked a hole inside ya."

He's joking, right? Not cool, I'm still all drugged up.

"Ed," I said as I rolled my eyes, "what the heck are you talking about?"

"When Dr. Miller inserted the needle into the umbilical sac, it caused a small hole in the inter-twin membrane."

"Oh, crap!" I said. "Is that something they can patch up?" I asked.

"No, and it's actually not as bad as it sounds, but it is something they'll need to monitor," he said, reassuring me.

"Katie and Lauren are safe—and so are you." He reached for my non-IV hand and gently kissed the top. "And that's all that matters."

For the first time since I had learned of the diagnosis, I let thoughts about the long path ahead sink in. The ablation surgery had just been one step along the journey, the most daunting step, perhaps, but still the first of many. We had weeks to go before the babies had even a remote chance of survival in the outside world. Twenty-three weeks. Even if they were born then, there was still just a slim chance that they'd survive and they'd almost certainly suffer from cerebral palsy or some other condition. Every week was critical. Every *day* was critical.

I stayed in the hospital overnight even though I was ready to go home. Everything was fine with me, but the doctors wanted to do another series of scans in the morning to check on the girls. Dr. Miller was performing another laser ablation surgery, his second of the week. Dr. Cooper came to the hospital to check on me and conduct the primary examination. I hoped, since he had delivered good news to us, before that he would be delivering good news to us again today. I waited nervously as he turned on the sonogram. He gently placed the probe on top of me and began to move it along the surface of my belly, obtaining various views. He stared at the two little images on the screen.

After a few moments, he said, "The good news, kiddo, is that both babies look like they're doing well, and Dr. Miller got a good separation of the placenta." He paused.

Oh gosh. Here comes the bad news. I braced myself.

"The bad news is, that during the procedure, a hole was created in the inter-twin membrane that separates the babies. See, sometimes Dr. Miller and his team do this deliberately as part of the treatment plan for TTTS. A septostomy, which is the term we use, is the intentional rupture of the septum that aims at balancing the amniotic fluid pressure in the two sacs leading to a correction of the placental circulation. In your case, I don't think it was their intention, but it's a small hole, and we had all hoped that the membrane would stay intact. But, it looks like one of the babies poked through this hole and started making the hole bigger. We all knew this was an issue yesterday but hoped that they would just leave it alone."

Well, nice going, girls. Of course, our girls couldn't let things be, they had to go fiddling with this inter-twin membrane thing. They were going to be mischievous meddlers those two.

"Katie and Lauren probably got into a cat fight—their first of many as sisters, I'm sure—and tore the membrane," Ed joked.

"Ed, really?" I turned and glared at him.

"So, what problems could this cause?" I said turning back to Dr. Cooper.

"Crystal, do you remember when you came here for an ultrasound a few months ago? We checked to see whether there was an inter-twin membrane? We confirmed that there was indeed a membrane and determined that you had mono-di twins—same placenta, different sac. Remember how it took us a while to see the membrane that separated the two amniotic sacs? Monochorionic-Monoamniotic twins don't have that membrane. So it's like they're sleeping together in one sleeping bag. There's no barrier that separates their umbilical cords. In addition to TTTS, the big risk is that their umbilical cords can become entangled or compressed, which can cause one or both of them to die."

More talk of dying.

"So, if the cords get tangled, there's a chance they'll die?" I asked.

Given the girls had already shown a desire to tear apart the membrane that separated them, I didn't think they could make it another ten weeks without doing something else risky in their now-shared umbilical sac.

"No, the cords will always get tangled to some degree. It's only if the cords get tangled in a certain way, or are pushed up against something, that there's a serious problem. We'll definitely need to deliver them early, as the risks of problems increase significantly after the thirty-second or thirty-fourth week of pregnancy because of their growing size." And then he let his other shoe fall.

"Kiddo, I want to have you admitted to the hospital sometime in the next week or so for monitoring."

"What? The hospital? For how long?"

"As long as we can keep the babies in—the longer the better."

"Are you kidding me? I'm only twenty-three weeks pregnant. It could be months before they are born."

"How soon can she be admitted?" Ed asked.

I shot him a dirty look.

"I'm thinking about the babies, Crys. I think we should do everything possible to ensure Katie and Lauren's safety."

"I know, Ed, obviously the girls' safety is our first priority," I glared at him.

This was unbelievable. We were falling further and further down the rabbit hole with these bizarre high-risk occurrences.

"Stay in the hospital the whole time? No breaks? For the remainder of my pregnancy, is that what you are saying, Dr. Cooper?" My voice cracked.

"Yeah, kiddo. I want to play it safe."

I didn't need clarification, but I asked anyway. I knew exactly what this meant. It still came as a shock. A long-term hospital stay would be excruciating on me and Abby, Ed—our whole family.

"So when are you thinking Crystal should go?" Ed asked.

"That depends on the insurance carrier's policies," Dr. Cooper explained. "Typically, they won't admit patients for in-hospital stays until twenty-five weeks."

"What? Why is that?" Ed asked.

"Just because there isn't a whole lot they can do until twenty-five weeks. We're monitoring to ensure everything is fine, but, if it's not fine, our only option is to deliver. Until the twins are at twenty-five weeks, there just isn't much chance of them making it if we have to go that route. You'll just need to take it easy and hope for the best."

Hope for the best? Are you serious? That wasn't exactly what I wanted to hear. I wanted a treatment that was more proactive than sitting around for a couple of weeks hoping nothing bad happened. And, the fact that some analyst had looked at the cost paid out to the hospital for a week of inpatient care and decided that any benefit conferred wasn't worth the cost was beyond frustrating.

Dr. Cooper signed my discharge paperwork, and Ed and I left the hospital. There was a week of waiting at home before I would go inpatient. The only thing I could do was stick to the regimen of bedrest as best I could even though Abby would want to play with me and jump all over the bed. Dr. Cooper's version of bedrest meant me literally staying in bed most of the day with allotted trips to the bathroom and to shower once a day. I even had to be in bed as I blow dried my hair and applied make-up. To kick start my bedrest party, Dr. Cooper sent me home with a care package containing all kinds of goodies—leg compression socks, a device to help with blood circulation, a stack of preemie magazines and a few hospital parking passes. Ed was going to need those. The only things missing were a bottle of bubbly and some chocolate covered almonds.

The news about our twins being Monochorionic-Monoamniotic—or MoMos, as they are also called—was disconcerting. I tried not to think about the whole umbilical cord entanglement. I tried to stay positive. We had survived the laser ablation surgery. Our little recipient, Katie's, heart condition had improved dramatically in just a couple of days. They'd still monitor her heart throughout the pregnancy, but both Dr. Cooper and Dr. Miller seemed legitimately impressed with her progress. We had beat one challenge—TTTS—and were now just dealing with the collateral damage that the laser ablation had inflicted.

One big battle down, but another one—a long, drawn-out one—was just beginning.

Okay, I told my unborn daughters. *I know that this hole y'all ripped in the membrane has put us at the highest risk possible for something to go wrong. But I have to admit, that if y'all made the hole so you could stay together in there—that is pretty darn cute. No, actually, that's the sweetest act of sisterly love I've ever heard. Now let's just pray nothing goes wrong.*

THE LIST

My restless nights at home continue and I dream of possible happy outcomes with my three daughters.

"Mama, Mama push me," Katie says as she toddles past me, her feet moving in tiny little strides.

"Mama, push me pweez," Lauren says as she pulls on my pant legs. We've just finished our picnic at the park, I look over at the lake and see ducks waddling into it. I'm holding Lauren's hand and we are walking behind Katie who's approaching the swings. Up ahead, I see Abby going down the spiral slide. "Okay, here we are," I say as I carefully place Katie into the high-back bucket swing, sliding her legs into each side. I pick up Lauren and place her in the swing next to her sister and then take a step back, giving them each a big push at the same time. I run to get in front of them and keep pushing. "Higher, higher Mama," Lauren says. She's smiling and giggling with Katie, who's laughing so hard. "I want to swing with my sisters too, Mommy," Abby says as she runs towards us. "Come here, sweet girl," I say as I pick her up and help her get balanced in her big kid swing. They are soaring high, shoes pointed up towards the sky, a slight breeze blowing their little ringlets. "Mommy can we go get ice cream after this, please?" Abby asks sweetly. "I scweem!" Katie says as she claps her hands. Lauren's face lights up with excitement. "Yes, my loves," I tell them. "We can."

To most people, a week of bedrest could seem like an eternity, but because I dreaded the check-in date so much, the days flew by. I spent as much time with Abby as I could—filling our days with music, books, art projects and lots of laughter. I tried hard to mentally and emotionally prepare myself for the weeks ahead. *How should I pack for a long-term hospital stay? What would I do alone all day? How would I keep myself entertained? How could I be separated from Abby for that long?* That would be the most heartbreaking part. One way to escape would be to sleep through it, but I knew sleeping all the time would depress me. With each passing day, my anxiety intensified. *Were the girls okay? What if their cords were entangled already? What if they keep entangling more?* I hoped I'd feel better once I was in the hospital and being monitored often.

After putting Abby down for her nap, I plopped down on the couch and opened up my laptop. I Googled "inpatient pregnant moms." A ton of hits popped up, some more helpful than others. I read stories about other moms' experiences—many of them emphasized the importance of having a plan. One mommy blog suggested decorating my nursery online—purchasing everything I needed, then hiring a professional organizer to set it up for me when I got home. Or they suggested starting a project. I could learn to crochet beautiful blankets and scarves just like my mom; I wished I'd taken the time to learn when she had tried to teach me in the past. I could make a list of all the starter materials I needed from the craft store, and then have Ed pick them up for me. Hmm... Nothing really grabbed my attention. I needed to give it some more thought. I closed the computer screen and set it down beside me, then grabbed a pen and paper and starting making a list.

Packing list for hospital stay:

- Comfy t-shirts
- Shorts
- Pants
- Pajamas
- Toiletries
- Make-up
- Blow dryer and flat iron
- Pair of slippers
- Flip flops
- Snacks and drinks
- Pleasure reading books
- DVD player and DVDs

For the next couple of days, I kept adding to the list, and it quickly grew to be more than just words on paper; it represented my life—my survival plan—for the next few weeks. I started adding not only daily necessities, but tangible items that would sustain me and remind me of our home. They were reminders of my existence outside the hospital—items I would find comforting.

- Pictures of Ed and Abby
- Countdown calendar

I read in some mommy blogs that a countdown calendar was crucial for mothers during an inpatient hospital stay. It would not only serve as décor on the bare white hospital walls, but become a meaningful ritual each day, marking the passage of time. Crossing off each day of a hospital stay marked a huge accomplishment. Each day enabled my babies to keep cooking. Each day meant less time in the NICU.

I added another item to my list that would make my hospital room homier, if that was even possible:

- Living room lamp

One night before bed, Ed grabbed my list off the bedside table. He shot me an incredulous look and said, "You're not seriously taking our living room lamp with you."

"You better believe I am," I replied. "Do you think I want to have only fluorescent lighting? The lamp will bring some life into the room and help me feel more at home. It's going," I asserted.

He read the rest of the list aloud: "Egg crate foam mattress, sheets, down comforter... Good Lord! Are you planning on permanently moving in? Want me to help you move the couch, too?"

"We don't know how long I'll be there, so I just want to make sure I'm comfortable."

"Okay, but why an egg crate foam mattress? I'm assuming they'll give you a bed, or is it BYOB—bring your own bed?"

I laughed and then explained.

"The hospital mattress is so firm that it'll hurt my back. I need to maximize the rest part of bedrest. If I don't manage to get some sleep, who knows...our babies might make an early appearance. And we definitely don't want that. So the egg crate foam mattress goes, too."

"Shower chair...I'm not even going to ask."

"Yup, that's right. I need that so I don't fall stepping into the shower. This ain't the Ritz. No walk-in showers were I'm going."

I knew there would be no shortage of staff and nurses around if I did need anything. At least that was comforting.

I put down the pen, set my list aside and rubbed my eyes.

"I can't believe I check in tomorrow. This week flew by. My parents will be here in the morning."

I'm not sure what we would have done if we didn't have family nearby. My parents offered to keep Abby during the week since Ed put in long hours at his firm. On Friday afternoons, he would drive to their place in the suburbs and pick her up so they could have the weekend together. We had planned that Ed would spend two nights at the hospital during the week. He would bring me dinner from the outside world, which would, no doubt, be an improvement over hospital fare. We would watch TV and hang out. It would give me something to look forward to as I would have fewer visitors during the week than on weekends. I knew I would look forward to the weekends the most—Ed and Abby would spend the days with me.

"I already miss my sweet girl." I was thinking it, and the words just slipped out.

"It'll go quickly. You'll see."

"Easy for you to say. You won't be on lockdown. I feel like Piper from *Orange is the New Black*."

LEAVING ONE CHILD TO SAVE OTHERS

On the day I was scheduled to check-in to the hospital, I woke moments before my alarm was set to go off. I felt large and swollen, but snug, under my soft jersey cotton sheets and fluffy down comforter. *Maybe,* I thought, *if I hide under the covers, no one will find me, and I won't have to go.* Too bad my gigantic baby bump made me like a hippo in hiding.

I felt Ed gently pat me on the arm.

"Just think," he said, "the next time you'll be back here, we will have two new babies."

If everything goes well, I thought. I smiled and nodded in agreement, but I was terrified of the possibility of returning home empty handed.

I savored every minute of my goddess shower that morning. That's what I called the glorious showers during which I actually got to wash and condition my hair. I shaved the top and the bottom of my legs. These were luxuries mothers of small children didn't usually get. When I returned, I'd be a mommy-of-three: two preemie newborns and a toddler. I might never have a shower longer than two minutes ever again. Well, until they all went to college.

I stepped out of the shower and onto the bath mat, the bathroom nice and steamy. I quickly blow-dried my hair and applied some body lotion, powder and lip-gloss. Mascara was a bad idea that morning, I decided. The goodbye was going to be brutal. I threw on one of my favorite pink shirts—a solid maternity keeper. It had carried me through my pregnancy with Abby, even at the end when I was feeling like a miserable beached whale plopped on the living room couch. I grabbed a pair of black yoga pants out of my drawers, slipped on some flip-flops and threw my hair in a ponytail.

From my bedroom, I saw someone standing in the doorway out of the corner of my eye. It was Abby, dressed in her pink unicorn pajamas, clutching her Snoopy dog.

Every morning she woke calling out, "Mommy, come get me," and then asked for milky. She was almost two. We had stopped nursing shortly after her first birthday, but she still found comfort in the cold milk that she drank from her sippy cup. Every day, without fail, the same two things: mom and milk—that was pretty much her whole world.

Leaving Abby was both nauseating and heart-wrenching. Even though it would only be for a few months' time, and she would visit with Ed some evenings and weekends, it was still incredibly painful. I had never been apart from Abby for more than a few days at a time. Our Paris getaway was the longest by far, and by the end of the trip, I was so ready to come back because I missed her so much. We had a strong connection—an immediate bond. The idea of leaving her for an extended period of time was like leaving a part of myself behind.

"Good morning, my love," I said to her.

"Mama," Abby said, extending her arms above her head for me to carry her.

I waddled over and scooped her into my arms. I kissed her cheeks and breathed her in; she had the scent of sweet baby lotion. Her skin felt so soft against my cheek. I stroked her hair and twirled her baby ringlets around my fingers. I had been dreading this moment for the past week and a half. *How was I going to get through this? How could I say goodbye to my little Abby?* I had tried, in the days leading up to my departure, to break it down in a way she would understand. But all she retained was that I was leaving. She was still just a baby—well a toddler—but my baby, and the reason didn't matter. She just didn't want to me go. I choked back tears.

I heard knocking, and then a few seconds later, the front door opened. It would be my parents arriving to take me to the hospital. Ed and my folks appeared in the bedroom doorway. I was on my knees, holding Abby so tight.

"Mama, come play," she pulled my arm.

"I can't play right now, sweetie. Remember Mommy told you, I have to go bye-bye for a little while." I began to cry.

"No, I don't want you to go bye-bye, Mommy" Abby yelled back, her eyes widened with urgency.

I glanced down, biting my lip so hard it bled a little. "You're going to stay here with Papa."

"Crys, aren't we all taking you today?" mom said.

"No," I sniffed. My dad handed me a tissue. "I was thinking registration and check-in might take a little while." I paused to catch my breath. "It might be easier for Abby to say goodbye here and not in a strange place."

"Yeah, that makes sense." My mom nodded. "Dad can stay with her here."

"Are you ready to go?" Ed asked.

"What do you think?" I snapped and burst into tears again. "I don't want to do this!" I yelled. I don't want to leave my little Abby. I don't want to leave home. And I don't even know how long I'll be gone. That's the worst part. Hell, I don't know if that's the worst part. It's all bad."

"Crys, she's going to be fine. We will take great care of her. Just keep reminding yourself that you're doing what's best for you and the babies. And even for Abby. Soon she'll have sisters. What's better than that?" mom said as she bent down and hugged me.

Ed came over and rubbed my back. "The monitoring will be so reassuring. Imagine if you were at home—with no monitors, undetected—if something went wrong. We could lose them in an instant." He paused, helped me up off the floor and then held me. He whispered, "We have come so far. I know we are going to get through this last part."

I knew he was right. I knew they were both right. I knew the monitoring of the babies' heart rates every few hours—in the hospital—would alert us if any serious complications arose. Their umbilical cords were already tangled since they were swimming in such close quarters; we just needed to make sure they didn't cut off their blood supply, which was what the machines would detect. I couldn't bear to think about losing my babies. I was frightened for their health. It made me terrified of saying goodbye to Abby too. I had so much guilt—leaving one child to care for another one, or in my case, another two. The guilt was all-consuming, like a parasite growing inside me. *Would Abby feel abandoned? Would she remember I left her?*

I didn't know the answers to these questions. I only knew that, as parents, we are often faced with extraordinarily tough decisions. How do we balance one child's needs against another's? When they are mutually exclusive? In my case it was obvious. Yes, it was going to be difficult, but I needed to be strong and acknowledge that other people—our family, friends, our support network—would be able to help care for Abby. Our family was expanding, and it wasn't just Abby I had to worry about anymore. I was the only one who could take care of these precious unborn babies.

I bent my knees in an attempt to get down to Abby's level, but I was too big to keep my balance. I was afraid I would topple over.

"Nope, that's not going to work," I said.

"Here. Let's try this." Ed picked Abby up.

I peered into her searching eyes. My tears re-emerged.

"Bye bye, baby girl. Mama loves you so much."

Tears were streaming down my face. I could taste the saltiness as they seeped into my mouth.

"I'll call you when I get to my room. Okay? We can FaceTime so Mama can see your beautiful face."

I hugged her tight for a long while to make up for all the hugs I wouldn't be able to give her during my solitary confinement. She wiggled a little, but Ed held onto her. I hugged them both and just leaned into Ed's shoulder. I finally let go, picked up my purse and walked over to my dad. I kissed his cheek and hugged him goodbye.

"*Que Dios te bendiga, mija*," he said. May God bless you, sweetie. "*Te quiero*." I love you. He kissed my forehead. My sweet father had immigrated from Mexico at the young age of eighteen; he lived on his own until he met my mom ten years later. He taught me Spanish as my first language when I was growing up, a life skill I'd always be grateful for, and we still often spoke to each other in our native tongue.

"*Gracias, Papa*," I whispered. "*Te quiero mucho*."

Ed handed Abby to my dad. We slowly walked out the front door. As Ed turned the key and locked the door behind us, I could see Abby through our big front window—the one she and our dog Charlie would lie in front of as babies and watch as our neighbors walked their dogs. She was out of Papa's arms and running towards the window; she banged on it to get our attention. She smiled and laughed—she probably thought I was coming right back. I blew her a kiss and waved goodbye knowing that I was doing the only thing I could do as a soon-to-be mother of three and not just one, but it still hurt.

PART 2:

THE HOSPITAL

MOVE-IN DAY

Dr. Cooper wanted me to check-in around 9:00 a.m.
I looked down at my cell phone. It was 9:02. Right on time. I wished we would've gotten stuck in traffic—anything to delay this moment.

"Crys, we're here," Ed said as he parked the car in front of the hospital valet.

"Okay," I responded, gazing off into the distance. From the hospital doors I could see the entrance to the zoo across the street. The gates had just opened, and the people that had been lined up down the street—as if it was a hot night club—began to flood in. The parking lot was filled with SUVs and minivans—parents applying sunscreen and bug spray to their children, loading pre-made picnics and coolers into their wagons and strollers. They were beginning their fun-filled day of animal sightings, jungle-gyms, train rides, ice cream cones and laughter. I would have given anything to join in the fun and be there with Abby. Almost anything, except for the well-being of Katie and Lauren. I snapped out of it. Even though a part of me believed despite all the dire warnings, I had to keep reminding myself that I could get through this pregnancy on my own without being a science project under twenty-four hour observation.

I stepped out of the car and took a few steps through the sliding glass doors. I was greeted by a hospital volunteer, a young guy maybe in his early twenties, wearing a brightly colored red vest that made it impossible not to notice him. He wore a nametag on his vest that read "Volunteer."

"Good morning," he said cheerfully. "Welcome. How can I help you?"

"I'm checking in as a patient in the antepartum unit." I said, setting one of my bags down on the floor next to me.

"Oh okay, let me arrange wheelchair assistance."

"No, I'm okay. A wheelchair won't be necessary."

"I'm sorry ma'am, it's actually hospital policy, for um…" he struggled to delicately state his next few words. "Pregnant moms that are hospital patients must be wheeled on hospital premises." He signaled to the guard standing next to a few empty wheelchairs who then wheeled one over to where I was standing.

Ugh, no thanks.

"Well, technically I'm not a patient yet," I told him.

I wasn't sure if the volunteer didn't hear my statement or if he just chose to ignore me. Either way, he stuck out his arm and offered me assistance in sitting down in the wheelchair. I handed my purse to my mom. As soon as I was seated, the volunteer took the break off of the wheelchair and began pushing me. We were off to the fifth floor antepartum unit.

I felt annoyed as we wheeled along. This mandatory ride made me feel as if I had already lost control of my actions. As far as the hospital was concerned, I was a liability waddling around. They were in charge from here on out, I was just along for the ride. It drove me—control freak in charge of everything—crazy to have to hand over the reins of my life to someone else.

We walked down the hallway and stopped and waited a moment for the elevators. I was here being admitted into a children's hospital. It all felt strange to me—to be wheeled around when I was fully capable of walking. I was neither sick nor injured. In fact, aside from dealing with the anxiety of my impending bedrest, I felt pretty darned good. Checking into a place for sick and injured people felt wrong.

The elevator opened up and we got in. We rode in silence for the five levels up to the unit. We stepped out of the elevator, and I instantly noticed a huge change in temperature. The temperature on this floor was sub-zero freezing. I rubbed my arms wishing I had pulled out my fleece from my duffle bag. As we wheeled down the hallway, we passed the hospital gift shop. It had two large, glass windows, and the display cases were filled with teddy bears, floral arrangements, tiny pink and blue cigar gum sticks and balloons. This is where visitors stop and buy gifts for their family members' and friends' new babies. Right after your baby is born, you get a flood of flowers, edible arrangements with the chocolate covered pineapple and bananas and soft fluffy stuffed animals that say "Baby's First Giraffe" or whatever. But then I wondered if it would be the same this time. *Would our friends and family stop at this gift shop and get our girls gifts?* I thought as I rubbed my stomach. My anxiety level rose, and I envisioned the first few days after the girls' birth and how different they would be than my experience with Abby. It tugged on my heart to think that my babies most likely wouldn't be coming home with me. They would be staying here in the NICU of this hospital in this arctic blast.

I checked in with the receptionist at the front desk of the antepartum unit. The hospital had gone digital since I had given birth to Abby. She handed me an iPad and directed me to fill out the extensive medical questionnaire. But I couldn't focus on reading the questions. I kept pausing and overthinking as if it were a difficult problem on a math test that I could skip and go back to at the end. I got to the last page and checked a bunch of boxes, then scribbled my signature on the iPad and dated it. *May 25, 2014.*

My life as an independent pregnant woman was ending, and my life as the long-term hospital pregnant mama was beginning. *Yup, I'm a long-term patient, checking in for God knows how long. The rest of my life.* At least that's how it felt.

"This must be how inmates feel on their first day," I said looking over at my mom.

"Only you don't have to wear an orange jumpsuit," she said with a smile.

"The thin blue gown isn't much of an improvement," I said.

We both laughed. One of the red-vested volunteers directed us to the waiting room and told us it might take a while to get a room since they had to wait for a vacancy in my unit. Meanwhile, I was still sitting in a wheelchair that could've been better used by someone else.

"Guess what?" I turned to look at my mom. "We get to hang out a bit longer." She smiled.

I stood up slowly and moved over to the waiting room chair. My mom pulled a crochet project out of her purse and started to work her needles. She was a pro. She had been crocheting since before I was a baby. She was making a baby blanket for one of the girls.

"Remember, you're going to have to make two of everything," I said.

"Oh, I'm already finished with the other one," she replied as her needles clicked.

I rummaged through my bag. I'd come fully stocked with trashy magazines and a stack of the newest chick lit novels. I pulled my phone and opened up Facebook. *Wait, why am I doing this?* I thought. Looking at other peoples' highlight reels was the last thing I needed. I closed the app and looked up to see Ed walking into the waiting area.

"Hey, did you get all checked in, babe?" he said bending down to give me a kiss on the forehead.

"Yup, now we just have to wait for a room to open up in my unit." I pushed the home button on my phone to check the time. "Which could take a while."

"That's okay." He smiled. "I have all day to wait with you, if necessary. I just got a nice email from Bruce, one of the partners at my firm. Everyone is being very understanding at work."

"They'd better be!" I laughed.

Ed eyed everything I brought from home and shook his head. "I need to take a picture of you with all your stuff. You look like you're moving into your freshman dorm room. Remember the chaos that day?" he snickered.

Ed and I had lived in the same freshman dorm at Georgetown but didn't know it at the time. Still, I knew exactly what he was talking about. I laughed as I remembered that day over a decade earlier. It had been a hot and sticky August day in Washington DC, and it seemed that all the college students were moving in that weekend. Just when it came time to haul all my stuff into the dorm, the elevators broke, making us—my parents and I—have to go up and down five flights of stairs about eight or nine times until we got everything moved in.

Thinking back on it, I never realized how hard it must have been for mom and dad to drop off their first-born baby girl at college. For the first time, we wouldn't be in each other's daily lives. I could see the parallel between my college dorm life—which now seemed so distant—and my time as an inpatient in the hospital. Move-in day in both instances was a mixture of emotions. Back then, I'd been nervous about living in a strange room and being away from home; I was annoyed about mundane things such as not being able to walk around in a towel after getting out of the shower for fear someone might barge into my room. There would be tight living quarters with little to no privacy, bad cafeteria food and a need to wear flip-flops in the bathroom.

Then, of course, there were the stark differences in the college life and inpatient life scenarios. As a college coed, life was relatively carefree. Sure, there was the occasional stress of midterms, papers and bouts of homesickness, but the interesting classes, diverse group of friends and free beer on weekends undeniably made up for it. None of these were life and death issues. And now, as a mom with a high-risk pregnancy, life and death seemed to occupy every thought. I thought about how each of my movements could impact my girls. *If I move a certain way will you girls get more entangled? Or compressed? Can you do Mommy a favor and just keep kicking constantly so I know you are okay?*

There I was ten years later sitting beside a wheelchair, waiting to move into my new hospital "dorm" room. I was a decade older—with slight wrinkles around my eyes, a few gray hairs and scars from my first C-section—and wiser. I knew that my time at Georgetown, that time away from home and my normal life, in a way helped prepare me for what I was dealing with. I was able to adjust to a new life before and I was confident that I'd be able to do it again, however much more heartbreaking it was this time. And I still over-packed, but thankfully the elevators worked.

During that college move-in weekend, of course there had been the annoyances—the frustration of the broken elevator and the August heat—but my mom, dad and I had so many memories of our last weekend together. We went to dinner on the Georgetown waterfront and then walked along it until we got to the monuments. We sat on the steps of the Lincoln Memorial with frozen yogurt and shared funny stories from my childhood, our time abroad in London and reminisced about the past. What I took away from that experience was that life would always be filled with frustration and grievances, but it was about making the most of what you were faced with. This belief is what would help carry me through my hospital stay. They may have dragged me kicking, screaming and bawling hysterically, but I didn't go there to cry in a room by myself all day. Oh, heck no. I wanted to bring to life and laughter to that sterile place. There would be social gatherings of some sort, good food, music and more.

My daydreaming in the waiting lounge ended when I heard my name.

"Mrs. Duffy," a beautiful blonde nurse said, "We have a room ready for you, Sugar."

CHAPTER 9

THE DORM ROOM

The blondie stepped behind me and took the wheelchair off the brake position. "Here, let me." She wheeled me passed the double doors, into the unit and down a long hallway.

Ed and my mom loaded up with my stuff. Each grabbed as much as they could, leaving one suitcase behind.

"Maybe they have a bellboy," said my mom.

"You're looking at him" Ed laughed.

"And a cute one, too," I added.

As we walked down to the end of the hallway, we passed several nurses' stations, a conference room and an operating room. We turned the corner and entered the wing, or pod as the nurses called them. My room was right across from the nurses' station. It was tiny, had one small window along the back wall, a door to the bathroom and a bed in the middle of the room. *This is it? I've been waiting all morning for a coat closet?*

"Welcome to your new room, hon," said the nurse. "I can help you get settled in."

"Oh no," my mom said, shaking her head in disapproval. "This room is awful, it's way too small. My daughter will be staying here for several weeks. We need a bigger room. I want her to be comfortable." She paused, eyes still scanning the room.

"Can you swap our room for a bigger one?" My mom looked directly at blondie.

"I'm sorry, ma'am," blondie said, tilting her head slightly. Her blue eyes widened so much that you could see the black eyeliner smudged under her eyelashes. "I was told this was an extremely high-risk case, and I wanted to make sure her room was near our station. I wanted her to be in close proximity to the OR in case of an emergency."

"Well dear, I appreciate your thought and safety concern, but because she's staying such a long time, we would like a bigger room. I'm happy to speak with your supervisor if that helps."

"She," "her," "this patient." It was so awkward with me standing right there. I was glad to have my mom as my advocate but couldn't stand feeling like a helpless patient.

"Yes, ma'am. I'll take you to the charge nurse and you can discuss the room assignment with her." Blondie left, my mom following behind.

Before she was out of sight, she said, "Don't worry, *mija*. I'll be right back. Don't unpack anything. We are moving to a different room."

"Oh man," I said to Ed. "I haven't even been here five hours, and she's already talking to the supervisor." I giggled and shook my head. "I hope the nurse doesn't get the wrong impression or think I'm going to be a problem patient." I giggled.

We looked at each other.

"I'm going miss you, Crys," Ed said quietly, the way he got when he tried to hold back emotion.

"It's going to be really depressing going home to an empty house. Without you or Abby, there's no reason to go home early," he paused, looking down at his cell phone. "There will probably be lots of late nights at the office."

"Or you can come here and hang out after work," I said. "It will be like junior and senior year all over again," I joked. "We can watch movies on Netflix and order late night pepperoni and jalapeño pizza from Domino's."

"That sounds nice," he said, perking up. "My plan is to come straight to the hospital after work a few nights a week. I won't even have to drive or worry about parking; I can just take the Metrorail. It picks up in front of my building and drops off at the hospital."

"It stops right across the street near the entrance to the zoo," I said.

"I know," he said, nodding his head. "I'm going to take Abby there all the time. Oh, and I can take your clothes home and do your laundry too," he offered.

"That'll be the first time you've ever done my laundry," I said and giggled. "Do you even know how?"

"Yes, I'm perfectly capable," he replied, playing at sounding annoyed.

The door flung open. My mom poked her head into the doorway. "Guess what?" She had a huge grin on her face. "We've got you a room down the hall that is literally twice the size! Come on, baby girl."

She was very proud of her victory. She helped me out of bed and back into the wheelchair. I double-checked the paperwork at check-in regarding the wheelchair assistance. It was in there plain and clear—every time I took a step on the floor, or really any other floor of the hospital, I had to use the wheelchair for assistance. It was a safety and liability thing. But, for me it was a pride thing. There we go again with the helpless patient act. I'm fine people, really. I'm pregnant not handicapped.

As my mom wheeled me back down the hall, we passed the nurses' station and turned right going past a few more rooms until we reached the corner of the hallway. We opened the door to room 582—my new home—for the next few weeks. It wasn't the Ritz by any means, but my new big, bright room made me feel like everything would be okay. It came equipped with a small refrigerator and a scale. In the back were three big windows that let a generous amount of sunlight through. Beneath the windows, there was a long bench with pull-out drawers for my clothes. The room smelled of Lysol, and the floors shined liked new appliances at the store. On the other side of the room were two sinks and lots of counter space on top of which there were a couple of hospital gowns folded neatly inside their plastic wrapping. The cabinets overhead came fully stocked with medical supplies. If anyone needed bandages, gauze or medical tape, I had them covered. On the far-right side, there was a desk, chair and small coat closet. A corkboard above the desk made the perfect spot for my countdown calendar. The bed was positioned in the middle of the room—there were no upgrades there, it was the same hospital-grade bed all patients used—with the various reclining positions and a remote control. The sheets were bleached white and stiff, in desperate need of scented fabric softener. There was a TV mounted on the wall opposite the bed. I'd be caught up on the Bachelor and Real Housewives—and just about every reality TV show—another plus. A small nightstand beside the bed had a little drawer with my own copy of the Bible and a prayer book. I was going to need those. Behind the bed was the monitor I had heard so much about—the one we would use to keep tabs on Katie and Lauren around the clock. It was an oversized, gray machine that rested on top of a wooden table. Big and bulky, it had lots of wires protruding in all different directions. A printer attachment would print the reports from the monitoring throughout the day. There was a tray where all the reports would be stacked neatly—making it easy for the doctors look at them when they did their rounds.

After I finished surveying my temporary home, I realized I was exhausted from being shuffled around. I just wanted to lie down and close my eyes.

Blondie entered the room. "I hope you like this room better." She winked at me. "Lunch is just about over, make sure you call down and place your order so they can bring it up to you. I'll give you a few minutes to eat, and then I'll come back and do your monitoring. Okay?" She was about to walk out the door when she turned around and stuck out her hand. "Oh, by the way, I'm Jenny." She smiled sweetly. I had never seen anyone look so glamorous in scrubs; her light blue scrubs accentuated her full-figured body. She wasn't big, but she wasn't petite either. The perfect in-between. She had a small waist and gigantic breasts, the kind that you just couldn't help but stare at, even as a woman. Her soft, curly blonde hair fell down to her shoulders, and she had full face of makeup.

"It's really nice to meet you, Jenny. Thanks for taking care of me today."

"It's nice to meet you too, sugar. And of course," she turned around, her curls bouncing off her shoulders as she walked out the door.

"She's sweet," I said as I turned to face Ed and my mom. "Marilyn Monroe meets Sweet Home Alabama. And gorgeous." I said.

"Oh, I didn't notice," Ed said sarcastically and shot me a guilty grin.

My mom looked down at her phone, then slipped it into her purse.

"Well, I'm gonna go, sweetie. Glad you are all checked in. Don't worry about Abby—she's fine. Very happy to be with her Gigi and Papa.

She bent down and hugged me.

"We'll come visit you in a couple of days," she said as she wiped a small tear trickling from the corner of her eye.

"Ok. Don't forget your crochet bag. You have to finish that blanket," I reminded her.

"Yup, I got it," she said and walked out, blowing me a kiss.

I turned to look at Ed, who was staring down at his phone, no doubt worried about the time—but also feeling guilty about having to leave me.

"All right babe, let's get you out of this wheelchair and into bed," he said.

"I'm fine. I can do it myself," I told him, and moved into the bed, even though I really just wanted to walk out with him. "I can't believe it's already noon." I gazed up at the clock on the wall. I had been so distracted by the logistics and the check-in process, I had forgotten about my sadness. As Ed slipped his phone in his pocket and started to say goodbye, it all hit me again. I'd soon be alone in this hospital room—without my family, without my baby girl—and trying not to constantly freak out about potentially dangerous cord entanglement.

"Don't leave me here, please," I told him. I started to sob.

"I'm sorry, sweetie. I'll come back this evening and pick up whatever you want for dinner. Then we can watch a movie together. It will just be a few hours. You're doing the best thing for the babies." he said, rubbing my belly and then bending down to kiss it. "We have to keep an eye on these two so they don't get into any more trouble."

Ed always had a way of phrasing things so that they weren't doom and gloom. He lacked theatrics, but in our relationship, I certainly made up for it.

We held each other so close; I never wanted to let go, much like with Abby that morning. Ed had been alongside me every step of this pregnancy. Each day after the diagnosis, he was by my side. His strength bolstered me and mine buoyed him. Would I be able to maintain my strength without him there with me? Reminding me that what I was doing *was* the best thing?

"Love you so much, my brave, strong girl. You are the most amazing mommy," he said, pulling away from me gently.

"I love you too, Ed."

And just like that, I was left alone. Alone in my room riding the wave of many intense feelings. It was all so emotionally draining and exhausting. But then it hit me—I'm not actually alone. I placed my arms around my belly, embracing it tight.

I'm not alone, I told my babies, I have you two girls with me. Every step of the way. Our journey together. And then, I realized that this would be the perfect time to tell the babies more about me and my life. What better way to pass the time then by chatting and getting to know one another? And so I settled on my bed and started to talk to them.

Being a mommy was a lifelong dream of mine, I started. I had yearned for it for as long as I could remember—long before I had even met Daddy. In preschool, I always chose the playing house center. I gallivanted in pearls and high heels, carting my baby doll in a stroller wherever I went. I spent my younger years babysitting my younger sister Melissa, and helping my Grandma Ita[1] babysit my younger cousins, Melanie and Caroline. Our family was very close; I saw my relatives daily. We spent every summer (even during the five years we lived

---

1   Ita comes from the end of the Spanish word *abuelita*, which means "grandmother."

abroad in England) at Ita's house escaping the sweltering Texas heat in the backyard pool—days of endless popsicles, splashes and laughter. Years before that, when my parents—you will know them as Gigi and Papa—went back to work after I was born, my grandparents took care of me every day. They were head-over-heels in love with their first little granddaughter and called me Cristalita. They took me everywhere on playdates and outings with their friends. The summer after I turned two, my Grandpa Ubaldo died tragically. It was utterly heartbreaking and so incredibly unfair—something that, over time, everyone in the family had to learn to grieve and accept in their own way. My Ita—while grieving—never let her shocking loss interfere with her endless love for her children and grandchildren. I absolutely adored her—in my eyes everything she did and said was perfect. I thought her life was both fascinating and inspiring.

Ita had grown up without her parents. Having lost her own mother in childbirth, she was raised by her grandparents in a small rural town in Northern Mexico. She was kind, generous, an extremely hard worker, a woman of strong faith and prayer and a firm believer in education. I remember she used to tell me to, "Earn all the degrees you can because no one could ever take that away from you." A degree, a prized possession that could never be lost. I learned everything I knew about cooking, cleaning and raising kiddos from Ita—all of the fast-paced multi-tasking involved. I'm not as great of a cook as she was, but, oh well. She could take care of us, cook, and clean all in one seamless effort. She was confident, strong and fierce, but utterly melted at any requests by her beloved angelitos,2 her grandchildren. And these are only the surface details of all that made up my Ita, Micaela Martinez. She was a beautiful person inside and out—not a day goes by since her death back in 2006 that I don't think of her.

I yawned, suddenly overcome by an overwhelming urge to lie down. *I will spend my lifetime telling you girls all about her, I promise,* I told the babies. B*ut right now, Mama needs to snooze.*

---

2   *Angelito's* is the Spanish word for "little angels," referring to young children.

I pulled my blanket out from my suitcase and lied back on the bed; I rolled over to my left side, my back to the door. I closed my eyes. I was almost fast asleep when a knock on the door awakened me.

MY ANTEPARTUM FAMILY

"Oh man," I grumbled. "Who is it?" I sat up groggily.
"Are you…" Before I could finish the sentence, the door opened.

"Hey there, Mrs. Duffy," a voice from the other side of the door spoke. A tall, handsome guy, in his mid-thirties stepped into the room. He walked towards my bed.

"Oh, my gosh!" he exclaimed. "I hope you don't mind my saying so, but you look like Selena Gomez." I smiled and blushed at the compliment.

"You know," he continued, "the cute little actress and singer that was going around with Justin Bieber. I'm so glad they broke up."

"Yes," I nodded. "I know the one," I replied. "And thank you, that's so sweet, and quite the compliment given that I probably weigh double her right now."

"I'm Paul." He extended his hand to shake. "I'm the head nurse for the antepartum unit."

His hair was perfectly styled; the gel had been meticulously arranged to position each strand of his highlighted bangs.

"Mrs. Duffy," I laughed. "That reminds me of my teaching days. That's, of course, what my students would call me. Well, half of them. The ones I had in my first couple of years called me Ms. Olguin and it stuck with them. The ones I had my last two years of teaching only knew me as Mrs. Duffy."

"Oh, sorry," Paul said. "Would you prefer Crystal?" He scribbled a note down on his clipboard.

"Oh, yeah, that would be great." I smiled at him.

Paul's eyes scanned my bags. "Wow! Look at you," he said, pointing to all my suitcases and belongings. "Planning on moving in permanently—eh?"

I laughed. "You sound like my husband."

"I'm just teasing. We're so happy to have you here in our unit. We are like a family; we take extra special care of our long-term patients." His attention now turned to my bed. "Your bedspread is gorgeous," he said, patting my brightly colored quilt—the same one I had had in college.

"Thanks," I replied. "Urban Outfitters, Georgetown, circa 2003."

"Love it," he said as he clapped his hands. "You must be so smart, a Georgetown grad," he said.

"No, not really, I'm just..." I struggled to find the right words. "I just work hard," I said. "And I did work my tail off to get into Georgetown," I explained. "But moving in here has strangely reminded me of moving into college. Minus the husband and kids part."

"I know how hard this must be for you," he said. He leaned in and patted my shoulder. "I've been reading your file. Twins, huh?"

"Yes, and double-trouble already, these two," I said rubbing my belly. And I told him the whole story of my challenging pregnancy. "I'm twenty-five weeks pregnant today." I could feel one of the babies kicking on my right side. They probably loved the attention.

Paul's jaw dropped. "You have been through a lot, my dear." He paused, as if trying to think of what to say next. "Well, you are in the best place you could be. I mean the Texas Medical Center—you have the very best at your disposal; it's the best place to be if you're in trouble." He laughed nervously. "We have to make sure those babies are safe and stay put awhile longer."

I nodded.

"Do you know about how long you will be here?" he asked as he looked down at my file.

"As long as I can make it. Although I know with Mono-Mono twins, the goal is to deliver around thirty-two weeks. But my plan is to take it one day at a time," I said.

"Yes, every day is huge," Paul said, his tone now more official sounding, like a doctor. "Every day the babies stay inside you can make the difference of weeks in the NICU." I kept repeating his words in my head over and over. "Each day in utero could make the difference of weeks in the NICU." It was mind blowing for me. Hear that girls, you gotta stay put for as long as possible.

He scribbled something down in my file. "Tell me if there's anything I can do for you. Special requests, furniture additions—we do have lounge chairs that are quite nice."

I perked up "Ooh! That would be great. Do you think you could get me one?" I said. "My husband, Ed, is going to be staying here with me three or four nights a week. I know he would really appreciate it."

"Sure thing. I'd be happy to track one down for you." He scribbled that down on my file too, then looked back up at me.

"Our nutrition specialist will be coming by your room later to discuss your diet during your stay with us and make some suggestions. Oh, and I almost forgot, my co-worker, Adrienne, will be coming by to say hello. She's the mama bear around here; she has a deep love for all of our patients."

Lots of visitors to welcome us, girls.

"In your file it says you are Catholic; Adrienne helps out the hospital's chaplain—part of our Catholic services in the hospital. So if you need anything—special prayer requests, she can do that for you." Barely remembering the box I had quickly checked on the form, I nodded my head in agreement.

"She's also working on organizing a support group if you are interested in participating."

I perked up again. Here was my chance, something that would help me stay social and pass the time. Maybe I'd make a mom friend who was going through the exact thing as me.

"I'd love to be a part of that, sign me up," I told him. "I'll double-check with Dr. Cooper—since I'm on pretty strict bedrest—but I'm sure it's fine as long as I'm wheeled down there."

Suddenly, I began to feel tired. "Well, thank you for all the information," I said. "It's helpful to know there are people close by I can call." I smiled hoping he would wrap it up and let me rest.

It had been a bit overwhelming—all the information, names and positions and duties. I'd probably forget half of what Paul went over by the time he left. I wanted to close my eyes and lay down.

We were interrupted by a knock on the door.

"Come in," we both said at once.

"Lunch delivery," said a girl in her early twenties, she wore a white apron that was tied in the front, and her hair was pulled back by a hair net; she was holding a cafeteria-style tray.

"Oh shoot! I completely forgot to order lunch," I said and glanced at the clock.

"Yes, we noticed you didn't order lunch, so we have to feed you, unless otherwise instructed," the girl said. She looked down her eyes surveying the food tray then back at me. "You are in luck—today it's a grilled chicken sandwich, potato chips, and a chocolate chip cookie."

"Yum, I'm starving; it's past lunchtime," I said, rubbing my grumbling belly. I know, sweet baby girls. I'm going to feed you. I bet y'all will love that cookie as much as your mama.

"Where should I put this?" she asked.

"You can set it down on the tray table here next to my bed. Thanks." I took the lid off of my plate and then placed my drink, plate and the assortment of condiments onto the table. I handed her the tray. I was literally salivating over the food, I was so hungry.

"Okay, I'll let you eat lunch," Paul said. "I'll come back and check on you soon."

"Thanks. Bye." I bit into my chicken sandwich; a little mayo dripped down my chin.

There was a quick knock and the door swung open again. Jenny came in wheeling a computer that was resting on a cart. In her hands were a big drinking cup and a small Dixie cup.

"I have your complimentary hospital cup filled with iced water, honey," she said cheerfully. "I also have your prenatal vitamin. I see that Dr. Cooper added it to the system here."

"Okay, thanks," I said, grabbing the plastic cup and taking a huge sip of water. I was parched.

"I was going to do your monitoring, but I see you haven't eaten your lunch yet, sugar, so I'll come back."

"Sorry." I took another bite of my chicken sandwich. "I've been getting distracted by visitors. But, yeah, that would be great." As I took a third bite, I discovered that the sandwich really had no taste. The first two bites were masked by my hunger. Even with the mayo, it was bland. There was absolutely no flavor or seasoning. I didn't know how someone could mess up a simple grilled chicken sandwich, but they had. Maybe some, salt, pepper, mustard and more mayo would have helped. Ooh, but there was a pickle! Pregnant lady loved her some pickles. Now if I can just get my hands on some chocolate ice cream, I thought. I wondered if I could talk the nutritionist into ice cream at every meal.

As I sat there imagining a gigantic bowl of marble slab ice cream, there was another knock on the door. *Again?* This place was busier than Grand Central Station. How was I going to get any rest? I reached for the potato chip bag. A tall, slender woman walked into the room.

"Hi Crystal!" she said in a high pitched voice. She had bright, fuchsia active-type scrubs that made her blemish-free, porcelain skin radiate. Her big, brown eyes were wide with excitement and her short black wavy hair parted to the side. "I'm Adrienne, the nurse manager. Hopefully

Paul's been by already." You must have been a cheerleader in high school, I thought. I knew very few people this friendly and excitable.

"Oh, hi there," I said, slightly mumbling. I was crunching down on the chips. "Yes," I nodded, "he was just here."

"Oh great! So, you are carrying twins—right?" she said, almost jumping in the air.

"Yes, I am," I said, taking a brief break from my potato chips. "There are two growing in here," I patted my belly.

"Oh, my goodness. But you are tiny for twins," she said sweetly.

"Thanks. I feel gigantic. I used to be small, in my normal non-pregnant state."

"I believe it," she said scanning me up and down. "How many weeks are you?"

"Twenty-five weeks," I answered proudly.

"Twenty-five and what?" she asked, rather peculiarly.

"Wait, what?" I was confused by her follow-up question.

"Here in the unit, we see each day as a huge accomplishment. Each day here makes a world of difference as far as the time your babies will have to spend in the NICU. So, twenty-five weeks and how many days?"

"I just turned twenty-five weeks today. We'll see how long I can keep these active girls in here. One of them tore a membrane, ya know," I joked.

"Oh, yes. Remarkable. I've been studying your file in the break room. I made a comment to a few of the nurses—we are all in awe. You guys have been through a lot. Your little twins are fighters for sure. And so are you!"

I always tried to stay humble when receiving compliments from others. But especially in the previous couple of weeks, all the kindness, support and encouragement really warmed my heart.

"By the way. Are they girls or boys?" she asked.

"Girls. Identical twin girls," I said proudly.

"Beautiful! So precious—what a blessing. And you have another child too?"

"Yes, a little girl, Abigail, she's twenty-two months. Almost two, in fact, I'll probably be here for her second birthday. Maybe we can throw a party here," I joked extending my arms to include my room.

"We can!" she said. I looked back at her confused.

"Yeah, you know, we can get the nurses together and throw her a little party here. That way you can still par-tay while technically still being on bedrest." She threw her arms in the air and did a little dance.

I laughed. "Oh, that's so nice of you to offer, we'll see." I leaned forward. "Do you think we could serve margaritas?"

She laughed. "I'll see what I can do." I clicked with Adrienne, from the first moment we met. There was something just so warm, maternal, and loving about her. It was like having one of my aunts right there with me.

Our girlfriend chat was interrupted by another knock. It was probably Jenny. I would need to get on the monitor ASAP.

Sure enough, Jenny reappeared. "Ya ready, honey? I really must get you on the monitor."

This would be my first one in the hospital. It had been over a week—the day after the ablation surgery—since we had done any kind of ultrasound or monitoring. I was eager to get some updates on my girls, or to at least see and hear for myself that everything was okay.

Adrienne leaned in and hugged me. "It was great meeting you, Crystal. Hang in there, Mama. And if I can offer you a piece of advice, treat your time here inpatient like a job. Make yourself a schedule, a routine, a list of things you would like to accomplish—and I promise it will make the days go by faster."

"Things to accomplish?" I asked, confused. I could accomplish a whole heck of a lot more beyond these hospital walls.

"You could start an electronic baby book for the girls, write a blog, scrapbook, finish ordering things you need for your nursery, journal about your experience here. These are some examples of things our other inpatient moms have done here."

"Oh, okay," I said. "That's a great tip, thanks."

"Of course," she said. "And hopefully you will join us for our support group, which will be meeting soon. I'll send the information to Jenny or whoever is working in the pod that day."

Pod, unit—all these terms the nurses said—I was still getting used to speaking in their code.

"Oh right," I replied, "Paul mentioned that. I'd love to meet other moms in my shoes."

"And you definitely will be able to there. If you need anything, please call me. I'll come back later to check on you and talk about our chaplain services." She handed me her business card, said a brief hello to Jenny, and left.

"Okay, sugar," Jenny said, adjusting her equipment. "Do you need to use the restroom or do anything real quick? I need a clear thirty-minute reading on the monitor in order to make my report to the doctors. So in other words, no bathroom breaks for at least a half an hour."

"I'm okay. Thirty minutes will fly by. I'll probably just play on my phone."

"Well, thirty minutes is the best-case scenario if both babies cooperate and stay on the monitor. You see, these fetal heart monitorings are critical. They're the reason you are here. They help us track the babies' heart rates and rhythms. They let us know how the babies are doing. Monoamniotic twins are considered extremely high risk because of the very real possibility of cord compression leading to death as a result of umbilical cord entanglement. Babies swimming around each other will do that."

Girls, I told the babies sternly, *did you hear that? You guys better behave in there. You may think it's funny to swim around each other but knock it off.*

"So, what is a good reading? Or, what are you looking for?" I asked, feeling dumb, like I should have already known this information.

"The average heart rate for a baby is between 110 and 165 beats per minute," she replied. "It can vary about five to twenty-five beats a minute. The heart range can change as the baby responds to conditions in your uterus. So when I say I need to see a good thirty-minute reading, it means that the babies' heart rates have remained consistently in the average range. If there's even the slightest peak in heart rate, it can indicate that the babies are in distress. So to be certain that they are not, we've got to keep you on the monitor to make sure the babies' heart rates come back down. If I have the slightest belief that the babies are in danger, I'll call the doctor on call. The OR is right down the hall, and they can deliver the babies in as fast as two minutes. That's why I wanted to play it extra safe and have you next to the OR." She winked.

I was completely blown away, not by the severity of the situation, because I had become used to that, but rather by how knowledgeable and helpful Jenny was. So much responsibility was being placed on her, well, all the nurses actually. Hell, I naively thought that the doctors would do my monitorings, like they did the ultrasounds. After all, wasn't that why I was there—for the doctors to keep an eye on me? Maybe not the attending docs but the residents—both of which I instilled lots of confidence in? But, no. Rather, these extraordinary, selfless people—nurses—were going to make sure my babies and I had the best chance to make it through this. They were going to keep us from harm's way. They had an unbelievably difficult task. They were my guardian angels on earth and in the hospital.

"Shall we get started, sugar?" Jenny said.

I took a deep breath. "Yes, let's see how these babies are doing." *Hang on girls.* I rubbed my belly.

It dawned on me how little control I had over what was happening in my growing belly. How little control *I* had over their destiny. I hadn't been able to stop the Twin to Twin disease, the septostomy, the Mono-Mono status—none of it. They were inside me and there wasn't a darn thing I could do to stop or prevent them from swimming around each other, further entangling their umbilical cords. It would also, from the outside, be undetectable to me. It drove me absolutely crazy to know there was not a damn thing I could do. I was so close to the girls, yet so far away.

CHAPTER 11

KEEPING THE FAITH

The warmed ultrasound gel used in Dr. Bill's office was replaced with the cold, hard-on-your-skin industrial slime that the hospital used. That damned ultrasound scanning gel. It smelled like rubbing alcohol and stung like aloe vera rubbed onto a sunburn. My sensitive skin was growing irritated from it. It had been smeared countless times over my stomach, and I assumed it would continue for the next few weeks. I couldn't stand the sight of it. What used to be something soothing had evolved to a dreaded chore. With the cold, gunky gel came the anticipation of something possibly going wrong. Every time the ultrasound probe was placed on my stomach over the gel, I would hold my breath and pray for the best.

Jenny pulled the scanner (or special stethoscope as I would come to call it) over to the left side of my stomach. I could hear a fast-paced bump, bump, bump.

"There's one of the baby's heartbeats," Jenny said as she fastened the stethoscope down on the spot and tightened it with the pink elastic belt over my belly. "Do you remember from the ultrasounds where the babies were positioned?" she asked, placing her hands on my belly and trying to feel around for movement to identify the position of the other baby. "Roughly?"

"Yes," I said, trying to recall the scan I had in the morning following the ablation surgery. "Baby A is on the left towards the bottom of my belly, and Baby B is on the right up top, closer to my side."

Sure enough, Mommy was right. As soon as I'd given Jenny the approximate locations, she was able to put the other baby on the monitor. The elastic belts were crisscrossed and pressed down tightly on my belly, making it hard to move at all.

"Ouch! That's a little tight," I said pulling up on the bed, trying to readjust myself to see if that would help.

"I know. So sorry, hon," she said, as she fastened the monitor down with an elastic belt. "Experience has taught me that the tighter I make, it the easier it stays on." She smiled. So basically girls, I told the babies, if I move, you guys move, and then the monitors move, which means we have to start this process all over again. So I'm going to try and lay perfectly still so we can get this done quickly.

"Aww. We have a pink belt and a blue belt," Jenny said. "Too bad we don't have two pink ones or a pink and purple. I know you're carrying girls." She tightened the second ribbon around my belly then gave it a gentle pat. "There. All done. Baby B is strapped down." She straightened my blankets and tidied up around the monitor, discarding some trash. "So do you guys have names picked out for the two?" she asked.

"Yeah," I said, trying not to move. "We've decided on Katherine Maria for Baby A and Lauren Elizabeth for Baby B."

"Wow. They are such beautiful names. Are they family names?"

"Katherine's middle name, Maria, is after my mom, who you met this morning. When Ed and I heard the name Lauren Elizabeth, we just fell in love with it. Our other daughter is Abby, Abigail Micaela, after my Grandma. She's almost two. I'm sure you'll get to meet her soon." I paused. "Oh shoot! I was supposed to call her after I was settled in."

"No worries. She's only two, so I'm sure she won't get annoyed that you forgot. I'll leave you to it. I'll be back in thirty minutes to take you off the monitor. I'll look over the reading, analyze it and make sure everything is okay before printing it out for Dr. Cooper to review. Doctors always make their rounds in the morning. Sometimes a resident will come around in the evening; it just depends. I may come in and adjust it before then if the babies move and get off, okay?" Jenny said as she grabbed my lunch tray.

"How can you tell if the babies have moved?" I asked.

"I can watch the monitoring session from my computer at the nurses' desk, so if there's any monkey business, I'll be watching closely."

"Oh, okay. Great." I felt relieved knowing there was always a pair of eyes on these two. Even if she wasn't in my room, I trusted Jenny and the other nurses on duty would be watching closely.

Jenny walked out the door and I picked up my cell phone from the nightstand. I was about to dial my parents when there was another knock on the door.

"Come in," I said feeling annoyed that I couldn't have a moment to myself.

A young brunette girl in her mid-twenties wheeled in a computer on a desk. "Hi, I'm Stacy, your nutritionist," she said. "I wanted to say hi and get your snacks and meals set up."

"Food!" I said enthusiastically. "Yes, let's do it, girl."

She laughed and launched into her spiel. "We offer a mid-morning snack and an afternoon snack. The mid-morning snack is scheduled to arrive between 10:00 a.m. and 10:30 a.m. and is usually a protein shake or smoothie with some type of fruit and peanut butter or jelly. The afternoon snack is usually veggies and hummus or cheese and crackers. Does this sound okay? Do you want me to make any changes?"

"No, I think that sounds perfect. I'll be well fed for sure." Or rather, you girls will. "One question: What kind of protein shake?"

"The packaged kind approved by the doctors. They come in different flavors: vanilla, chocolate, and strawberry."

"Sounds good. Do they rotate them so you don't get the same flavor every day?" I asked.

"Yes, I can make a note of that in our system." She quickly typed a note. "Can you think of anything else that you need?" She looked back at me.

"Three meals and two snacks a day. That's more than I get at home. I'm good." We are good.

"Okay, great. If you think of anything you need, my extension is 1033 on your phone there." She pointed to the antiquated landline phone on my nightstand. "Enjoy your stay here with us," she said as she wheeled her computer back out the door.

"Enjoy your stay" was something I'd expect to hear at a resort at Riviera Maya or the Bahamas, not a hospital. Still, I was grateful for how nice everyone had been to me; it was a relief. At least everyone was understanding and quite accommodating.

Before anyone else could come in, I grabbed my phone. I was dying to hear Abby's voice.

My dad answered. "Crystal! *Hola mija.* How's it going? How's your room? I heard you got a nice upgrade."

"Yeah, it's nice. I'm doing okay. Been busy so far."

"Busy, *querida*?"

"Yeah, between my string of visitors and my monitoring—which I'm actually on now, never a dull moment."

"Visitors already? Que sociable, my little social butterfly. Already making friends in the hospital."

"Several of the hospital staff members have come by to welcome me."

"That's great, *mija*. I'm glad they're treating you well. They'd better! Abby's doing well. We had a snack, and she's watching a movie— Frozen, she picked it out. Later I'm going to take her to the park down the street from us."

"Frozen again? Oh, bless it. That's great. She'll love the park." As I said that, I teared up. I could hear giggling in the background, her sweet laugh. It made my heart ache. I just wanted to hold her, to kiss her soft cheeks and put her little hands in mine. I remembered a time I'd taken her to a park once when she was about fourteen months old. It was a gorgeous fall day, crisp and about seventy degrees. The leaves had just started to fall. We arrived at the park and she was glued to me; she didn't want to go in.

I squatted down so we were eye-to-eye. "Sweetie, what's wrong? Don't you want to go play?"

She shook her head. "No, I just want you, Mama."

Her words melted my heart. She was my firstborn. Her clinginess never bothered me. I genuinely loved having her around me all of the time. It was that connection, that strong bond; we were one and the same person. When I was growing up, I was never a big fan of running around in the dirt or crawling through tunnels, but I'd always enjoyed the swings. So I scooped her up and pretended she was an airplane flying in the sky. She loved it and laughed hysterically. I took her over to some cool looking lounge-chair swings. "Abby, try these. I think you will like them." I placed her gently in the swing and fastened the buckle. No sooner had I started pushing her, she was soaring like an airplane with the biggest smile on her face. She said, "Again, Mama, again!"

"Do you want me to put Abby on the phone?" my dad asked.

I paused. I would have loved to talk to her. I would have loved to ask how her day was going, how she was enjoying her time with Papa. But at that moment, I just couldn't bring myself to do it. I feared that if I heard her sweet little voice, I'd completely lose it, putting my little ones at risk during the monitoring.

"No, that's okay. We can FaceTime later tonight. Make sure she doesn't watch too much TV. Engage her in diverse activities, play with her—blocks, puzzles—or read books."

"Don't worry about us here—just take care of those gemelitas." My twins. My precious little girls.

"I will," I sniffed. "Okay, I've got to go. The nurse is coming back to put me on the monitor." I lied so I could quickly get off the phone.

"Okay, sweetie. We love you."

"Me too." And I hung up.

Phew! *Deep breath. Try to keep it together.* I rubbed my eyes. As I reached for a tissue from my bag I heard someone else at my door.

"Come in," I said as I blew my nose.

"Hi, honey." It was Susan. She was holding some balloons and two pink teddy bears.

"Are you okay?" she asked as she came over and sat on the end of my bed.

"Oh yes, fine, just missing my little Abby," I said, trying to smile.

She came over and hugged me tight for a few minutes. Tears trickled down my cheeks. I didn't say anything and neither did she. We didn't need to. It was extremely comforting having someone who understood, not my exact position, but about being inpatient and away from a family. She slowly pulled away, rubbing my back gently.

"I brought you some little gifts," she said, handing me the two teddy bears. They were incredibly soft. She tied the balloons to the end of my bed.

"That's a great spot for those." I broke a smile.

"When you checked in, dear, you mentioned you were Catholic, and would be interested in being contacted by a chaplain or some of our volunteers. So here I am. This is another one of the hats that I wear around here."

"Oh, yes." I perked up, wiped my nose with a tissue and placed it on my lap. "I would really love to set up a time once a day, or once every few days, to have someone come pray with me. I'm not sure how long I'll be here, but I want to remain strong in my faith. I need someone to help me keep my faith going, even as I get through some more difficult times in this pregnancy."

"Of course," she said and nodded. "We can definitely arrange that. Do mornings work for you?"

"Yes, I'm pretty much free all the time, except when I'm hooked up to the monitor, like now, but even then I can still talk."

There was a knock on the door. It was Jenny. *Thirty minutes already—that's good*, I told the babies. *It means you girls behaved and didn't move too much.*

"I'm sorry to interrupt y'all," Jenny said as she slowly unfastened the monitor belts. "You are done with your monitoring, sugar. And I got a clear thirty minute reading from the babies, so you can have a break and a nice long chat."

"Oh great," I said scratching at the indentations the belts had left on my stomach. "Everything look okay?" I asked.

"Yup, both Katherine and Lauren look great—nice strong, healthy heartbeats."

"Oh, wonderful," I said, again, feeling so relieved."

"I'll be at my desk if you need anything, darling," Jenny said as she walked out again.

I turned to look at Susan. "This is great news. These monitorings are a big cause of my stress and anxiety. They are the whole reason I'm on long-term bedrest in the hospital."

"Oh yes," she nodded. "Indeed they are. Crystal, would you like to talk, maybe tell me a bit about yourself?" she asked.

"Sure, I'll start from the beginning," I said. "Do you have an hour?" I joked.

"As a matter of fact, I do. I have as much time as you need. I'm here until 7:00 p.m."

As I shared everything Ed and I had been through, every painful little detail, I began to feel as though I were chatting with an old friend. Susan was warm, compassionate and caring. She gave off such a peaceful and calming vibe. She listened to me as I went through everything, pausing to cry and then laugh. She patted my shoulder when I sobbed and joined in laughter when I told a joke for comic relief. She always seemed to respond with exactly what I needed to hear.

"I'm trying to have a positive attitude and keep strong in my faith while I'm away from home, but it's so hard," I said.

"Your strength will carry you through this pregnancy and delivery just as it has carried you this far. And it will be passed onto your girls as well. They are going to be strong and beautiful, just like their mother," she smiled.

Her words stayed with me. The idea that my physical and emotional strength, something intangible, would be passed down to my girls was invigorating. If I could have picked anything, any trait for my girls to inherit from me—beauty, brains, humor—I'd pick strength. College buds, some of the people who knew me the best, always joked and called me "apex predator," the top of the food chain. Our good friend Mike once told me that I was the nicest, sweetest person in the world, but if you mess with my family—especially my kids—I will mess you up. I smiled to myself as I thought that my girls could also have this big personality trait.

It was nice to be able to talk with someone freely who was not a doctor, family member or someone who knew me before all this. I wanted compassion and kindness without the pity or judgment that went along with it. And actually, almost every person that Ed and I had told about our situation had expressed those things—caring, kindness and compassion. We had received countless offers to bring us food, meals, babysit Abby, run errands. These unexpected acts of kindness warmed my heart. But why then, did I manage to remember the one or two people who had responded harshly? "Bedrest? I'm jealous. That sounds nice. I'm always so tired from working, I would love bedrest." This comment occurred in a conversation with a mom friend from Abby's playgroup the week before I left for the hospital. Another woman had commented, "Wow, hospital bedrest, that would suck so bad. I don't know what I would do if that happened to me. I'm glad everything went perfectly for both my pregnancies and deliveries." Really? I'd thought. Do you have half a brain? Or heart? I never spoke to this woman again, and later discovered through the grapevine that she was suffering from severe post-partum depression and refused to seek help for it. It wasn't her fault, per se. But perhaps, because I was in such a place of deep pain, I was vulnerable and felt that I would be judged or looked down on for having had such a terrifying series of bad things happen. Did she smoke, do drugs or drink during her pregnancy? Did she exercise too much? There are so many normal twin pregnancies, what did she do to make her twin pregnancy so high risk? For that reason, Ed and I decided never to publicly announce anything on social media, but rather to groups of people we felt should know and people we knew would support us. I had tried in the previous few weeks to toughen up and not care how people reacted to my situation. It didn't matter what they thought about it or what they would do in my place. It mattered what I was doing to strengthen and empower my girls.

We had so many people in our lives who loved us. They were ready to help and couldn't wait to meet Lauren and Katie. I decided to stay positive and strong and focus on that.

Susan and I talked well into the afternoon, through the afternoon snack delivery and cleaning service. I shared some of my deepest fears—including things I had continued to question in my faith. The main question was: *Why?* Why me? Why my babies? Why are there some women who are allowed to breeze right through pregnancy and deliver baby after baby, and I must suffer? These were the things we discussed—things that made my faith even stronger.

Susan told me all about her role as one of the chaplains. She told me about the resources available to me through family services—including an indoor playground on the ninth floor.

"No way! A playground upstairs?" I said, excitedly.

"Yes, and it has a beautiful view of the zoo. You might even be able to see some animals on a clear day."

"Abby will love that," I told her. We had made countless trips to the zoo, always arriving early in the morning, so we could make the feeding hour for the giraffes. If you went between 10:00 a.m. and 10:30 a.m., you could feed the giraffe lettuce. Abby delighted in feeding animals.

"Crystal," Susan said as she wrote a note to herself, "I'm going to sign you up with children's services. They will bring you a plastic tub of toys—ranging from puzzles and coloring books to tea sets—all age appropriate. You can keep them in your room for when Abby's visits.

They will switch them out every week so she can have new toys to play with."

"Aww. That's wonderful. Thank you so much." My eyes began to fill. I wiped away a tear with my finger.

"Oh, I almost forgot," she pulled out more goodies from her tote bag, "here's a calendar, prayer book, rosary and a Bible for you to keep."

She reached out to me.

"If you'll give me your hand, please join me in a prayer." After we finished our prayer, Susan hugged me and headed for the door.

"I'll see you soon, Crystal. Good luck settling in and God bless."

"I will. Thank you."

I was happy that I'd been able to find some peace—that I was able to talk to, and confide in, someone I'd just met. I had always known that, if I kept strong in my faith, God would carry me through this. It was just a matter of having an awesome presence around to remind me. With a sense of spiritual tranquility and peace washing over me, I drifted off into a peaceful sleep.

CHAPTER 12

ROUTINE JOB

I felt a warm touch on my shoulder, then a tender kiss on my cheek. As promised, Ed had returned to spend time with me.

"Hey, sweetie. I'm back, how was the first day? I brought you dinner," he said.

"Oh, already? What time is it?" I said, sitting up groggily. I breathed in the aroma of Thai food.

"Almost 6:30 p.m."

"Oh man," I said and yawned widely. "I was out for over two hours. I was wiped."

"Long day at the office?" Ed said while setting the to-go bag on the tray table in front of my bed. He switched on my lamp.

"Actually, it went a lot better than I thought it would. I mean, I thought about Abby every few minutes, but I had lots of visitors to distract me."

"Really? Like who?"

I went through the day's activities—everyone I had met—my antepartum family—Paul, Susan, Stacy, and Jenny—and my first impressions of them. "Paul is hilarious, he's someone I would do happy hour with, and Susan is the sweetest—she really does feel like family, and someone I can confide in spiritually. For a split second I thought ahead—of us being past all this—the girls born healthy and us coming back for reunions or to have lunch and catch up with everyone."

"That's great." Ed said, pulling plastic tubs holding our dinner from the bags. "I was worried when I didn't hear back from you during the day. I

wasn't sure if they had taken you to get an ultrasound or for monitoring."
He licked his fingers. The sauce had spilled out of the tubs.

"Oh, actually," I said, "the nurse does the monitorings herself in my room. I don't have to go anywhere. She tracks the babies' heartbeats and reports her findings to the doctors. She calls them immediately if there's an irregularity."

Ed set down plastic forks and knives. "Were the readings okay?"

"Oh, all good," I said.

"Thank god. I brought us Thai food."

"I know," I said, smiling. "I smelled it right away."

We removed the lids of our piping hot pad Thai, set them aside and were just about to take a bite when the door swung open.

Jenny popped in. "I'm leaving for the day. My shift ends at seven. I'll debrief the night nurse who will be here until 7:00 a.m. She'll do your next monitoring, probably around 6:00 p.m. or so." She smiled at me.

"Okay." I swallowed the noodles I had crammed into my mouth. "Will I be woken in the middle of the night for the next monitoring?" I said.

"Yes, the doctors' orders say every six hours. If you want to discuss any changes or adjustments, the doctors usually make their rounds a little after 7:00 a.m."

"Okay, good to know."

"Do you need anything else, sweetie?" Jenny walked over to the large whiteboard in the room and erased her name, which had been written there in black Expo marker. "I'll actually see you in the morning. I'm back on this pod."

"Oh, good. I'm not going anywhere," I said.

Jenny walked out, curls bouncing as she closed the door behind her. I shoveled more noodles into my mouth. Ed's eyes widened as he watched.

I wiped my mouth. "I didn't eat much lunch and slept through my afternoon snack."

Our dinner was from Joy Garden downtown near Ed's office. This place was a favorite of ours. Abby and I sometimes met Ed for lunch there on Fridays. I teared up as I remembered the last time we were there, just the three of us, months before any of this started. Abby ran between the tables, waving at customers, completely mesmerized by the large fish tank. She loved animals of all kinds.

"I miss my Abby," I said. Tears welled up in my eyes.

"I know, sweetie," Ed said. "This is so hard. Did you talk to her this afternoon?"

"Earlier. She was perfectly fine. She's having so much fun with Papa."

"Isn't it better that she's so young she won't remember any of this… and one day this will all be a distant memory for you."

Not so sure about that, hubby, I thought

"Oh, right." I lied. I bit into my egg roll.

As we finished our dinner, Paul appeared at the door.

"Paul?" I said surprised. "I was just telling Ed about you."

"All good things, I hope." He placed his hands on his hips.

"Of course." I smiled.

"I have a present for you, my dear." He opened the door wide. In the hallway sat a large purple leather lounge chair. It reminded me of something out of a Dr. Seuss book—whimsical, bright and oddly shaped. And very used.

"It looks comfy and loved." I smiled with approval.

"I know it's kinda funky, but I got it from the pediatric unit, peds, as we call it. I gave it a test drive. It's super comfortable."

"Great! We'll take it." I said, motioning for him to bring it in. I turned toward Ed and said, "You're welcome."

"I'm sure it will beat sleeping on the window bench seat," Ed joked.

Paul put the chair between my bed and the window bench.

"Thanks so much," I told him as he turned to leave.

"No problem," he said. "I'll see you tomorrow morning. I'll try and swing by after the doctors' round. Susan is organizing an antepartum support group for the moms on our floor. Would you like to attend?"

"Yes, Susan already mentioned it to me. I'd love to get out of my room and meet some other moms."

"We'll double-check with Dr. Cooper and make sure it's okay. Sometimes the doctors get huffy puffy if they're not in the loop, but Dr. Cooper's cool, so you should be fine. I'll have a nurse bring you a wheelchair, and we'll get you down there."

Oh geez, again with the darn wheelchair. My bedrest wasn't categorically the worst or the strictest. There was partial bedrest and complete bedrest, and I'd say I was somewhere in between. A girl I went to high school with, Sally, had had to be on bedrest for pre-term labor prevention and her doctor didn't even allow her to get up to use the restroom. She had to use a bedpan and have hygiene services performed by hospital personnel. Bless her heart, as we say in the south. Really. I knew this was great in comparison to that. But still, schlepping around in a wheelchair wasn't something that felt right to me.

"Have a good night, you two," Paul said as he walked out.

Ed moved to the bed and sat beside me. He leaned in to massage my shoulders. I surrendered to his touch. "That'll be really good for you. You can meet other moms going through this inpatient ordeal. I'm sure you'll make some friends."

"I'm actually really looking forward to it," I said. "It's like I have a structured schedule still—a routine, places to be, people to meet up with."

A semblance of normalcy with adult interaction sounded heavenly. *No offense, girls,* I told the twins.

I'd given this some thought already. I didn't want to lose my mind, which seemed easier said than done considering everything I had on my plate. I planned to get up every day, shower, get dressed, put on make-up and fix my hair like I would in my normal life. I wouldn't let this become a free-for-all, an excuse to stay in my PJs all day and watch endless episodes of *Days of our Lives* on daytime television. I'm a driven person, I'd treat this as a job I'd excel in. And it really *was* a job. I was incubating two babies and doing a pretty damned good job, at least I thought so, especially considering everything we had gone through to get here. And this wasn't just the past few days, or the past few weeks, but the rocky start from day one. I made it through believing I was having another miscarriage right after I'd discovered I was pregnant, and I would get through this too. I wasn't about to let this experience drive me One Flew Over the Cuckoo's Nest. I refused to become a prisoner of my own mind. I would create a schedule—a daily routine—and perform my job. This would help me pass the time, keep me sane and carry me to the healthy delivery of my babies. I was feeling positive and upbeat, and the next morning I would kick-start this job by going to my first meeting. I drifted off to a deep sleep.

Despite drifting off feeling positive about things, my dreams never let me escape the horrors of my previous miscarriages. That night was no different.

The casino was dimly-lit and smoke-filled, the din of the slot machines made it difficult to hear each other.

I leaned over the green felt craps table. "Oh, come on, please get me doubles," I said.

"Blow on the dice for good luck," Ed said.

"Any day now," said Clay, our college friend.

"All right, all right. It's my first trip to Vegas. I hope I have beginner's luck."

I rolled the dice but got a four and a three, not the doubles I was hoping for. "Darn it!" I yelled. I had only wagered twenty-five dollars, so I hadn't lost too much.

"Better luck in the fantasy football draft," teased Clay.

"Come on, Crys, I'll buy you a cocktail at the bar," said Ed.

"I can't drink, remember?" I threaded my arm through his.

"Shucks, sorry. I keep forgetting," said Ed.

"It's a good thing you're pregnant during this Vegas trip, because otherwise you would probably be living it up a little too much right now."

"Oh please, I'm a mommy now—soon to be mommy-of-two. A few cocktails wouldn't exactly make me a scene from *Girls Gone Wild*."

"I know. I'm teasing," he said, smiling.

"Besides," I said, tugging his arm, "It's kind of fun being the only one of our friends not drinking because I get to remember every detail of everyone making a clown of themselves."

"Speaking of which, let's go meet up with the rest of the group," Ed said and steered us towards the casino entrance.

We walked down the long hallway and made our way outside onto the strip. The fresh evening breeze felt so nice after the stuffiness of the casino.

"Hey Ed," I whispered into his ear as I wrapped my arm around his. "I'm scared. This is our third pregnancy, what if something goes wrong again?"

We stopped in front of the club where the rest of our group was hanging out. "I'm hoping to have a healthy baby," I continued, "but with the crapshoot of pregnancy, who knows what's in store for us? We've tossed the dice and are hoping for a winning roll."

"Ha, fitting since we are in Vegas," Ed said. "But seriously, Crys, don't worry, and don't think about what happened in Hawaii. Two completely different pregnancies, and this time you are several weeks further along. You're almost at the end of the first trimester, and then we will be in the clear." We pushed through the door and stood together in the crowded foyer. We were going to have to push our way inside.

"I know," I said, and smiled down at my stomach. "Look at this little bump."

And then, from the corner of my eye, I saw something crawling on the floor. It was a solid, black ladybug.

"Oh, that's weird, "Look, Ed, down at the floor there in the corner."

"Oh wow," he replied. "That is weird."

Suddenly, I was overcome with a powerful feeling of dread. "Let's go," I said pulling Ed's arm.

"What's wrong, Crys?" he said.

"Nothing, just a bad feeling. Like that's a bad omen or something."

"Don't be silly," he said. "Come on, everyone's waiting on us to get into the club."

The music was blaring and the dance floor was packed. Strobe lights flashed in all directions as people crowded the bar getting rounds of shots for their friends. The room was hazy with cigarette smoke.

"Dance, Crystal," my friend Claire said, taking my hand and making my arm sway.

"No, not tonight, thanks," I said.

Something suddenly was not right. My stomach hurt. I had to go to the bathroom.

Oh my goodness. Please not again, I prayed. *Please, please, God, not again.* I'm felt something dripping onto my dress' underwear. I sneezed from the smoke and knew the drip had increased.

My eyes surveyed the crowded room desperately. In the far-right corner, I saw a dimly lit sign marked "Ladies' Room." I ran over and swung open the door, then closed it and didn't even bother to lock it. I sat down to pee and everything rushed out.

Oh my god! What the hell is wrong with me? I thought desperately. *How can this be happening to me again?*

Passing the blood made me nauseous. I leaned over and chunks of undigested food propelled into the air. I tried to get up and fell. I got up again, grabbed some toilet paper and wiped my face. When I looked into the toilet bowl, I knew it was too late.

"Oh God, please no!" I screamed.

The bowl was filled with blood which made it hard to distinguish what was what, but at the center was a definite blood clot.

Ed barged into the restroom. "Crystal, I was looking—" he started, then screamed, "Oh god!" as he saw the blood and vomit. "Are you okay? I'm calling an ambulance. We need to get you out of here."

"It's over." I told him. "Our baby is gone."

As I pushed away the nightmare away, I realized I was shaking. We'd been through so many horrific losses.

"What's wrong?" Ed asked leaning over to my bedside. "Bad dream?"

"Yeah," I said, rubbing my eyes. "I don't want to talk about it."

That miscarriage had happened just nine months earlier. Right before we left for Paris. I grieved in the months following the loss. Ed and I talked about it, cried about it, prayed about it; everyone had gotten over it, and moved on—Ed, our families. Everyone but me. My third pregnancy had brought me so much excitement and joy. But the happiness was so short-lived. What the hell was wrong with me? How could this have happened again? I wanted to scream, cry, run and hit something. I wanted to turn back time, or better yet, fast-forward through this painful nightmare. But I couldn't change a damned thing. All I could do was to ride in despair in the back row of the pain train.

Everyone had their opinions and unsolicited advice. Miscarriages were so common! They were our bodies' way of getting rid of a problematic pregnancy, a fetus that wouldn't survive. Was this supposed to help me? I wanted a concrete reason. Was it something chromosomal or my own failure to eat enough folic acid? But the truth was, the reason didn't matter. The bottom line was that that child was never meant to be.

There was a brief knock on the door, and then a small red-head walked in holding a stack of freshly folded towels. I glanced at the clock—it said 11:30 p.m.

"Hi, I'm Nancy, the night nurse," she said. "I'm sorry I'm late checking in. I got pulled into doing another patient's IV which took longer than I thought, and then another mom on the unit went into labor. Crazy night. There must be a full moon."

"Sounds like it." Ed said looking up momentarily from the briefs he was reading.

"Let's go ahead and get started on your monitoring."

"Okay," I respond groggily, still half-asleep. I sat up on the bed and rolled up my t-shirt, waiting for her to gel up my belly and begin.

"You'll have to forgive me because I'm new to antepartum," she said. "I used to be in pediatrics—I mean, I'm trained to do this…it's just been awhile."

"Okay, no problem," I said trying to break a smile.

Just please let this go well, I prayed, *so I can have some reassurance that my babies are doing well. That I need not worry.*

She started fiddling with the monitor, and after several minutes, finally flipped the on switch. She stepped back and scrutinized the machine, then the floor, then turned to me and asked, "You don't by chance know where the elastic monitoring belts are, do you?"

I leaned over to the side of the bed and pulled out the wooden drawer underneath the monitor. I grabbed the two belts and handed them to her.

"Oh, thank you," she said. She sounded relieved.

"No problem, I saw Jenny put them there."

I pointed to the spots on my belly where the babies had been in the earlier monitoring in hopes that it would help Nancy out.

After a few failed attempts, she paused.

"Well, it seems the babies have both moved. Let's see if we can track them down."

There were only two babies in there and my womb was only so big. You'd think there couldn't be that many places they could hide. Wrong. There seemed to be an endless amount of angles and positions, ways they could twist and contort so they wouldn't be picked up by the monitor. Every time Nancy would find one baby and strap the belt tightly on that spot, the baby would move. Track, locate, tie-down and move; track, locate, tie-down, move. Over and over again.

"Are you kidding me?" Ed finally said. He was beginning to get frustrated with this process. It was midnight and we still hadn't succeeded in finding either baby for longer than a minute. "Do you want to call and get a nurse to help you?" he asked. "This is going to take all night and Crystal needs to rest and not be stressed."

I turned, looked at him and whispered, "It's fine."

"She can't seem to track down the babies," Ed said. "Maybe they can do an ultrasound or something."

"I'm doing the best I can, sir," Nancy replied.

"I know you are, but it's late and it's been a really long day. We want to help you find the girls the fastest way possible so we can all be at ease." Ed can be quite persuasive in his arguments—both in court and at home—a trait that can be quite annoying at times. But when he pleaded his case, it worked.

"I can go see if one of the other nurses in the unit is free and can assist," Nancy replied.

About ten minutes later she returned with another nurse, Lindsey, who was fair-skinned with beautiful long, dark hair. Lindsey was a seasoned antepartum nurse, and we were hoping that, with her on board, we could get the babies on the monitor and keep them there for a bit. Lindsey meticulously placed the monitor on every square inch of my belly in hopes of picking up the slightest trace of a heartbeat.

"This is so weird," she finally said. "I'm usually able to find babies on the monitor right away."

"It's as if they don't want to be found," Nancy interjected.

"Our little Thelma and Louise," I said, looking down at my belly.

"Well, like it or not, girls, ya'll need to be monitored," Ed said, speaking to my belly. "That's the whole reason we are here."

"I'll keep trying," Lindsey said. Thirty more minutes passed before Lindsey was finally able to track both babies down and tighten the elastic belts extra snug; she used rolled up towels and washcloths to keep the belts from moving.

"There, this should hold them in place," Lindsey said as she adjusted the towels to keep the monitor at its precise angle. I was a funny sight lying there, belly exposed, with colored elastic belts wrapped in different directions around my belly.

Nancy came back into the room after thirty minutes. "The twins looked good," she told us, and then added, "you should really get some rest before your next monitoring session."

Geez thanks, Captain Obvious, I thought.

"What time is that one?" I asked, yawning.

"2:00 a.m."

"2:00 a.m.?" I asked, anxiously. "That's in less than two hours."

Ed looked upset. "This is so ridiculous," he said. "Can't we skip the 2:00 a.m. monitoring and do like a 6:00 or 7:00 a.m. monitoring so Crystal can get closer to a full night of sleep?"

Lindsey shook her head. "The schedule currently says to monitor every six hours, but since the last one got started late and took a little longer than expected I can't push back the next monitoring. You can discuss it with Dr. Cooper tomorrow."

"Geez okay," I said. "I'm going to try and get some shut-eye in before our next monitoring. See you in a few hours."

CHAPTER 13

WE'RE ALL IN
THIS TOGETHER

I felt soft patting on my leg. I was lying on my left side. My blankets were all twisted.

"Excuse me, Mrs. Duffy," said a soft voice. I opened my eyes and saw an African American woman in her mid-forties standing over me.

"Hmm, what?" I said groggily. "Why are you waking me?"

"I'm sorry, miss. I need to get your temperature and blood pressure."

"Oh, all right," I grumbled.

I propped myself to an upright position and opened my mouth so the woman could insert the thermometer. She then cuffed my arm and started taking my blood pressure. She worked quickly and efficiently.

"Thank you, goodnight," she said as she walked out the door.

I wiggled back down onto my side, twisting and turning to reach that optimal, most-comfortable position. My fan was propped up on a chair next to the bed. I leaned over and cranked it up to the highest setting. My eyes closed.

And then the light was switched on.

"Mrs. Duffy," Nancy called.

"Are you kidding me?" I said. "That other lady was just in here taking my vitals."

"Oh Janet, yes," Nancy said. "Actually, she was here about an hour ago."

"Can you turn off the light, please?" I moaned groggily. "We can use my lamp instead."

"Oh sure," she said. "That's a good idea. I'll need a bit of light to do your monitoring."

My head was throbbing and my throat was dry. I reached for the water on my nightstand and took a big gulp, then applied some ChapStick. *This must be what prisoners feel like,* I thought.

"I'm sorry," Nancy said as she grabbed the ultrasound gel from on top of the nightstand. "I know you just want to sleep, but I really need to make sure the babies' heart rates are okay. Then I can report my findings to Dr. Cooper. He should be by in the morning. That's when the attending and residents make their rounds."

"Good to know," I said nodding off again.

To say Nancy had a hard time finding both babies' heartbeats would be an understatement. Just as she located one baby, the other would move and throw the whole thing off and we had to start over. Were the girls plotting against us deliberately? Trying to keep me up all night? *So is this how it's going to be, Katie and Lauren?*

My eyelids were droopy and my eyes felt like sandpaper. I'd nod off to sleep, and then the monitor alarm beep would startle me, indicating that one of the babies had evaded the monitor once again. Don't want to be tracked, huh? I told them. Please, just do this for Mommy so we can know you're okay and I can get some rest.

Exhaustion and sleep-deprivation were not what I had envisioned with hospital bedrest. I needed to be rested before the babies were born. Otherwise, how would I stay awake through all those night feedings and diaper changes when they arrived?

It felt as if I were running a marathon, and instead of starting the race slow so I would have the endurance to finish strong, I'd started the race sprinting; I'd be drained at the end. During the day, my room had been a flurry of activity. People in and out, each one needing something from me, whether it was taking my vitals, asking questions or reminding me to eat. It felt as if every other person who'd popped in had to make a comment about food or eating. I would definitely need to start allocating some time each day for a solid nap. Maybe I could write a "Do Not Disturb" sign and Jenny could post it outside my door.

Ed, who I had almost forgotten about since he'd been able to sleep through the last monitoring, was awake. He gave me a kiss on the cheek and then hopped into the shower.

There was a quick knock on the door, and Jenny walked in.

"Good morning, sweetie, I'm back in this pod today. Can I get you anything right now?

"Sleep," I said half-snoozing.

"Bad night?"

"Lots of interruptions—seemed like all night long."

"Oh no, I'm sorry. You can go back to sleep if you want. If your breakfast tray comes, I can just set it down on your table for you."

"Oh thanks, but I'll wait," I said. "I want to be awake when Dr. Cooper stops by."

"I saw them walking down the hall doing rounds," Jenny said. "They should be by soon."

There was a knock on the door. "Speak of the devil," I said and pointed to Dr. Cooper as he entered my room.

"Good morning, kiddo. How's my favorite patient doing?" His voice reminded me of Humphrey Bogart in *Casablanca*. If anyone else called me a kid, I probably would have gotten annoyed after a while, but with Cooper, it was just part of his charismatic personality. He approached my bed, scrub cap on, looking sharp. Who looked that good at 7:00 a.m., and in a scrub cap to boot? A modern-day Humphrey Bogart.

"I'm okay," I answered.

"You settling in? Everyone treating you alright?" He winked at Jenny.

"Everyone has been great. Just some problems with my monitoring schedule," I said, yawning.

"I was awake most of the night," I said, rubbing my bleary eyes. "As the night nurse tried to find the babies' heartbeats, they moved around a ton. I think they were practicing their dance steps. I'm exhausted—I feel, and probably look, like a zombie from *The Walking Dead*.

"Oh, do you guys watch that show on AMC? So good!" Cooper said.

"I do normally," I said, "but I don't think I need the stress of roaming zombies and gruesome bloodshed while trying to keep calm on bedrest. It may put me into labor—an unintended consequence of zombie-watching." I gave a tired smile.

"Yeah, better stick to those daytime soaps," Cooper joked. "But, seriously, to address your concern, I completely agree. You need to rest as much as possible, which means getting a good night's sleep. I can change your monitoring schedule to every four to six hours during the day, and if everything looks good, you can have an eight hour stretch of uninterrupted sleep at night." He scribbled a note and handed it to Jenny. "How does that sound, kiddo?"

"What about the person who takes vitals in the middle of the night? Not cool. Is that really necessary?" I added.

"We can make a note in your file for all nurses and techs to do 'cluster care.' It means they come in together at the same time and get everything they need from you at once instead of interrupting you at different times."

"That sounds really great," I said. I yawned and stretched my arms over my head.

"I'll have Jenny write out a timeline and schedule for your monitorings so you can plan your day."

"Yes, a schedule would be so great. I'm trying to establish a routine and keep a schedule during my time in the hospital." I perked up.

Dr. Cooper turned towards me. "Crystal, I think you are going about this with the best attitude. I wish all my patients were as positive and upbeat as you. Sometimes I'll walk into patients' rooms in the middle of the day and the lights will be off, the shades shut and they'll be staring at the TV with no sound."

"Oh, man. How depressing. I definitely won't let that happen." I vigorously shook my head. Cooper nodded his head in agreement.

"Also, speaking of which, I have a small request. Is it okay for me to attend an antepartum support group meeting this morning? Susan organized it with all the moms on our floor. Paul can arrange a wheelchair pick up."

I felt like a teenager asking my dad for permission to go to the cool kids' party. With Dr. Cooper keeping such a close eye on me, I felt I needed to run it by him to make sure I wasn't exerting myself too much.

"Yeah, that sounds fine. Remember, a little walking around is good—keeps your blood flowing." He paused. I'll check in on you later. Call if you need anything. Jenny will take good care of you—she's one of our best nurses," he said, patting her on the shoulder.

"Try to relax and enjoy. "Dr. Cooper is the best," Jenny said. "He's my OB too. He delivered my daughter what now seems like a lifetime ago."

"Aww, that's awesome," I gave him a thumbs-up.

"Thanks, kiddo. See you soon. Hang in there." On his way out, he noticed my countdown calendar hanging on the wall. "Love this. What a great idea. You can mark off each day. You're doing great, by the way." He shut the door behind him.

"Okay, sugar, here's your prenatal vitamin." Jenny handed me a small, white cup with a little white pill inside. I popped it in my mouth and then sipped my water.

"I'll work on typing up your schedule, and I'll check in with Susan about the meeting time." She scurried out and twenty seconds later there was a loud tap on the door.

"Breakfast," a young guy holding a tray appeared.

"Oh, shoot! I forgot to order breakfast. I'm going have to set a reminder on my phone."

Ed had just emerged from the bathroom showered, shaved and dressed for work.

"Ed, want to split my bagel?"

"Sure. Then I gotta run. Early meeting this morning." He took a quick bite, which was basically half the bagel. Two bites and it would be gone.

"I'll miss you tonight," I said with a long face.

"I know. Me too, but I'll give you a call to check on you later." He grabbed his briefcase.

"Okay, love you," I said.

"Love you too, sweetie. Stay strong." He left, closing the door behind him.

Finally, some peace and quiet, I told the girls. *Let's have a cuddle.* I rubbed my tummy.

My room had cleared of the morning hustle bustle. I relished in the moments of peace. I took my time eating what remained of the bagel, carefully spreading the cream cheese. Then I picked up the spoon and finished the fruit salad and oatmeal. And then I had a chat with the babies. *You girls must be growing,* I told them. *Y'all are famished this morning. What do you think of all this? Crazy, huh?*

I clicked on the TV and leisurely watched the end of *The Today Show,* then slowly climbed into the shower using the rails and my shower chair. Afterwards, I threw on a nicer outfit—some maternity jeans, and a blue button-down top. I didn't want it to seem as though I had just rolled out of bed when I met my new antepartum mama friends. I powdered my nose and applied mascara and shimmery lip gloss. As I stared at my reflection in the mirror, I almost didn't recognize myself. My stomach had expanded to the point where my shirt buttons were about to pop off. My nose was spreading wider, and my cheeks were as chubby as a breastfed baby. *Well,* I told my reflection, *here's to hoping all returns to the way it was before.*

I unpacked some more of my things. With strict hospital bedrest, I was really supposed to be in bed at all times, only walking around to shower or use the restroom. I was being more mobile than I probably should have been. *Okay, girls, no crazy flips or entangling,* I told the twins as I looked in my purse for the photos of Ed and Abby I'd brought. I taped them on the corkboard next to my calendar. The room was beginning to look more like a dorm room—cozy rather than cold and institutional. And for that reason, I was glad I had lugged all those things from home.

Paul interrupted my decorating. "Hey, sweetie. I have your cool ride." He wheeled in a wheelchair. "Hop on!"

"Only if you'll take me for a super-fast spin down the hall," I told him. "I'm ready for a little excitement around here!"

"Oh, trust me," Paul said, "there's enough excitement going on with those twins of yours. You just can't see it."

"That's the problem. Isn't it?"

I sat gently into the wheelchair and placed my feet up on the footrests. We headed down the long hallway, passing several different pods, the vending machines and more patients' rooms. When we arrived at the big conference room, Paul wheeled me in.

"Hi Crystal!" Susan exclaimed from across the room. She ran over and hugged me tightly, like she was one of my aunts and I had just arrived to family reunion. As expected, the room was full of pregnant women; about twenty patients crowded around the conference room table. A young woman sat at the head of the table resting her arms on a guitar.

"I'm so glad you could make it," Susan said with a smile so big you would have thought I had just handed her a thousand bucks. "We're still waiting on a few more, and then we can get started." She touched the musician girl's shoulder. "This is Caroline, our music therapy intern. We are lucky to have her until the end of the summer."

What the heck is music therapy? I wondered. It sounded cool.

"We thought it would be nice to get all the antepartum moms together and have Caroline lead the group in some discussion. And hopefully serenade us with her beautiful self-written musical piece."

"Yeah, that sounds great," I replied. And it really did. I scanned the room for an empty chair. The place was packed. It was fully surrounded by pregnant women who, just like me, were stuck there because their babies were at risk. A few more women trickled in behind me.

"Here you go, sweetie, please take my chair." Susan said motioning to the spot right next to Caroline. I carefully got out of my wheelchair and squeezed into my seat.

From my angle, I could see that the faces of the other women bespoke misery—water works, stares and silence. *Well, this is a fun crowd*, I thought. Had some of these women been on the ward so long that the stay was wearing on them? And would that be me soon?

Perhaps their pregnancies had been more stressful than mine, I told myself consolingly, though that was hard to imagine. Or maybe they were just uncomfortable from the growing pains of the third trimester. Maybe they were just over being pregnant altogether. I could relate in many ways, but I hadn't reached the point of woeful resignation that filled the room. The women carried their unhappiness in their body language, in their pained expressions and their resigned demeanors. Two of them were so lost in their depression, they were quietly crying in a corner of the room. A couple of others were sobbing more openly; a few scowled while others sported their resting bitch face. Several ladies, I realized with a shock, were wearing hospital gowns with nothing on underneath. I even caught a glimpse of some squashed butt cheeks from behind. So incredibly awkward. I quickly averted my eyes.

I despised those lightweight, airy and revealing gowns; they reminded me of surgery.

Jenny had given me a gown when I checked into my room, but it was still folded neatly on the counter. There was no way I was going to wear *that* as a uniform every day. That, I could imagine, would truly make me feel like a prisoner. There were other women in their pajamas and bathrobes and some in their husbands' oversized baggy T-shirts and pants.

I detected a strong scent of body odor. I might have been the only one in the room—besides Caroline, Susan and Paul—who had bothered to shower that morning. My sense of smell was particularly heightened by the pregnancy. I scanned the room on the verge of gagging when Caroline looked over and said, "Crystal, would you like something to drink? We have snacks too. Sweet Susan baked cupcakes."

"Just some water would be great," I said, even though I was thinking, *How* about a little air freshener in here?

She handed me a cup of water which I downed in ten seconds.

And then, she stood up and addressed the group. "Welcome, everybody. We really appreciate you all coming to our first antepartum unit support group. I'm Caroline Scott. I'm a twenty-three year old grad student at the University of Houston studying music therapy. I'm originally from Ohio, but I'll be in Houston for a couple more months as I complete my internship with the hospital."

She paused to take a sip of water. I could tell she was nervous; her hands were slightly shaking.

"A little bit about music therapy: it's used mainly in the health profession, a therapist, like myself, assesses the needs of each patient and then provides indicated treatment such as creating, singing or listening to music. It can be incredibly helpful to provide an avenue for communication and can be helpful to people that are finding it difficult to express themselves with words.

How cool, I thought, *to find a creative outlet in music to express yourself.*

"I thought we could go around the room and have everyone introduce themselves, maybe say your name, how far along you are in your pregnancy, and if you would like, please share a little about your experience. Afterwards, I'd like to do a musical exercise. This is

Jewel," she said holding out her acoustic guitar, "named after one of my biggest inspirations. I'll play for you guys."

Her speech was accentuated by a thick Midwestern accent. She was a tiny little thing, just a little over five feet tall. Her long light brown hair was braided and pulled to the side; freckles dotted her nose. She reminded me of a former student, Meredith Walker, who was a cheerful member of the band and a hard worker.

The introductions started at the opposite end. As we went around the room, no one spoke more than their name, and only some shared how far along they were in their pregnancy. They offered the information stoically and robotically: Kim—twenty-six weeks; Sarah—nineteen weeks; Jennifer—twenty-nine weeks. It really did make us sound like inmates. Then it was my turn. I thought of following suit and just continuing the two-word response, but then I thought that maybe I was brave enough to share my story first. *It will help others going through the same things I am.*

"Hi everyone. I'm Crystal Duffy," I said with a warm smile. "I'm twenty-five weeks pregnant with identical twin girls." I told them about my sweet Abby at home with my parents. Then I shared my story. "We were told terrifying things—that both babies might die, or only one would survive. We had surgery that corrected this problem, but it resulted in another big problem. My twins became Mono-Mono twins—extremely rare—which puts them at a higher risk for cord entanglement. That's when my doctor advised me to come here."

The faces of the mommies on the front line lit up and they leaned in to soak up every detail. One woman had been napping and perked up as I told my story. The women offered sympathetic comments: "Oh no," "Wow," and "I'm so sorry."

Another mom jumped in. "I'm pregnant with Mono-Mono twins too. I just got here last week."

I was excited to have met someone (or rather lots of someone's) who could understand everything I was going through. My words encouraged a woman named Kim, the twenty-six weeker, to tell her story. Because she was older, getting pregnant was huge for her. She had almost given up on having children. Like me, she carried identical girls but she had received the news that they were Mono-Mono twins in week ten. She had carried this fear through nearly her entire pregnancy.

And then several other ladies shared their stories. All were a little different, but each one ended in that little hospital conference room. Both Caroline and Susan seemed visibly touched by the group sharing and the dialogue that was sparked. Some ladies broke into tears as they talked about how hard it was to leave their other children at home and how desperately they were missing them. That got me every time. Thinking about missing my little Abby made my heart sore. I wondered how she was adjusting to life without Mommy. Did she cry in the morning when I wasn't there to greet her? Did she cry at night when I wasn't there to comfort her? Did she wonder what happened to me?

The pain in my heart was unbearable, but somehow, being amongst the pregnant mommy brigade lifted me up. I knew I was not alone—the room was filled with women who shared the experience of enduring risky pregnancies. Each of us had different experiences that connected us and made us one—one entity of heartbreak, one entity of strength. We would be there for one another throughout our hospital stays. Then, one by one, our paths would diverge—giving birth at different times, being discharged and leaving our world that teetered on the fragile precipice of life. And hopefully, we'd all depart with bundles of love—happy endings. But that was just it: we never knew day-to-day how our stories would unfold—whether the things we risked would play out in unimaginable ways.

But, for right then, we were all in it together.

CHAPTER 14

TOGETHER AGAIN

I'm definitely a people person, so I wasn't surprised at all
that I quickly took to Caroline. She was a breath of fresh air in
the hospital—young, vibrant and brimming with positive energy.
Caroline seemed perfect for the job of music therapist. She was a
compassionate listener, even at such a young age. Though she had
no "life experience" per se, and of course didn't know exactly what I
was going through, she was empathetic. She seemed down-to-earth,
with her long wavy hair—usually in a side braid—and her own sense of
style. And her musical talent was out of this world. She could strike up a
melody and put lyrics to it in a matter of minutes. She considered Jewel,
her guitar, to be her child.

"She comes with me everywhere, even bars and restaurants," she told
me, clutching the guitar close. It always made me laugh when she'd
tell me her adventures with Jewel around Houston and the people they
would meet. Me and Jewel could be a funny column.

Caroline and I were complete opposites. I was a bit of a diva, a
fashionista and didn't have a musical bone in my body. Even so, we
quickly became very close. Our group meetings continued at least
once a week, sometimes twice if there was interest. I became friendly
with Kim because of our twin connection. Our antepartum group would
spend time sharing our passion for arts, music and traveling; we shred
all the hopes and dreams that we hoped to instill in our children one
day. Caroline joked that she loved our talks because she was gaining
so much valuable information that would benefit her in the future—
both personally and professionally. In addition to our chats, we would
harmonize together and do a variety of musical exercises. At times we
would analyze imagery and themes from classic oldies such as Elton

John or the Beatles; other times we would re-write the lyrics to popular songs from Adele, Shakira and of course Jewel.

Other times, when there were just a few of us present, we would play games and create songs using Mad Libs. We would see who could come up with the funniest one. I relished making up songs; it reminded me of being a girl in grade school. It was care-free, and there was no right answer. You let your creativity flow and see what sounded the best.

On one occasion, Caroline asked us to close our eyes and envision ourselves in the most peaceful place on earth.

"What sounds do you hear? What is the weather like? What does it smell like? How does it feel?" she whispered to us softly.

I envisioned the Pacific Northwest—either Washington or Oregon. I was surrounded by towering pine trees and everything was brilliantly green; a waterfall spilled into a trickling stream. It felt like a scene from *Twilight*. I even had my own Edward. At our next meeting, Caroline surprised us with personalized CDs of our favorite relaxing sounds. Mine featured the trickling water I loved. I played it in my room as night settled in. It sent me far away from the four white walls and the flashing, beeping medical devices. I could almost feel the spray of the waterfall on my face. I wondered if my girls could feel it too.

So this is perhaps what Mommy needs to play for you girls to settle down at night, I told the girls the first time I played the CD. Just like most things with babies and small children, sometimes the CD would work in calming their in-utero kicking matches and other times it didn't and I'd have to try a variety of other things—belly massages, lavender oil, humming, chanting—in hopes that one of them would have an effect on the monitorings. Sometimes they did. Sometimes they did not.

One afternoon, Caroline addressed the group, "If anyone is interested in doing their own project, you could journal your feelings and then we could make a song. I could help you put it to music. Afterward, we can record it and I'll make you a CD." She paused and looked right at me. "It's a tangible memento to take home with you, so you can reflect on your emotional journey bringing your babies into the world."

My family and friends had tried to reassure me by saying things like, "Don't worry; in a few years you won't remember this time," "It will be a distant memory that you had to live through once" or "You'll brush it off afterwards." Only, they were dead wrong. How could I ever forget my time in the hospital? How did anyone simply forget months of their life spent alone and scared shitless? I made the best of the situation with distractions from Caroline and music therapy but it was still hellish.

After my first miscarriage, it seemed like everyone, including Ed, had moved on from the loss except for me. I was the only one still grieving for that baby that could have been ours. Everything in our tiny apartment reminded me of our would-have-been baby. I wanted to move to a different place entirely in hopes that my sadness wouldn't follow me. But we weren't able to do that, at least not right away, so I took an old shoebox and placed all the baby related items I had lying around in it. My first and only ultrasound picture taken at six weeks, some onesies and baby socks I'd purchased, a tiny baby blanket, a cute monkey lovey and my own childhood confirmation pin. One day, I would pass the pin to our baby; if we had a girl, she could put it on her charm bracelet. This overly-stuffed box got pushed to the top shelf of our walk-in closet and was buried there for several months. In the time between the miscarriage and pregnancy with Abby, that box served as a reminder of what I had survived and what I had to look forward to one day. In moments of grief and sadness I would take it down, sit on the floor of my closet and look through the items, clutching each one and crying as I held them in my hands. It helped me work through that pain to know that I had the items in a box and didn't have to carry that grief with me constantly. It was there when I needed it to be, and when I didn't, it was stored away where it wouldn't constantly weigh me down. I knew this CD, this song would be like my baby box—a reminder of what I lived through and survived in order to bring my babies into the world. I was okay with that. I knew that, even after I was discharged, I would remember every friggin' detail about being an inpatient—every sound and smell—and everyone who was a part of my journey. I was intrigued by the idea of creating a song that would capture my deep emotions during this time.

When the group meeting was done, I approached Caroline. "Hey, so I think I'm interested in creating a musical project," I said. I paused, waiting for her reaction. "With your help of course," I added.

Caroline's face lit up. She was probably thinking, Great, I can write about this in my dissertation: How I helped a high-risk pregnant girl.

"But I'm not sure exactly what to write about," I confessed.

She put her hand on her chin to think. "Hmm," she said. "Have you journaled while you've been here?"

"No." I said. "I haven't... I find it too painful to write down everything I'm feeling. I get upset and start to cry."

"Let me ask you this," she said. "What's been the hardest thing about being in the hospital?"

I knew in an instant what that one thing was. It had nothing to do with being bored, alone or homesick. It didn't bother me that the medical team poked me with needles, administered medication and still checked my vitals every few hours despite Dr. Cooper's adjustment to the schedule.

The most excruciating thing about being here was the possibility of losing my twins at any moment, and this fear was tied equally with missing Abby—the baby I was away from while I was pregnant with two babies we still hoped and prayed would live through all this. This song—the first one anyway—needed to be about Abby. My yearning for her, my precious, angelic, easy-going mini-me. She was our miracle baby. She was the baby I once thought I would never have. Clever and focused mixed with funny and silly, she was the perfect amalgam of Ed and me. Abby was everything to me. Her every move—her every word—was my whole life. I was devastated that I was missing out on her day-to-day life: daily prayers, alphabet letters in the bathtub, morning walks with Charlie, library story time, Friday lunches with Daddy, afternoon park play dates. I missed all of it. I was stuck in the hospital freaking out about my babies while simultaneously missing out on her life. I thought about her every minute of every day. Had she eaten lunch? Something other than just milky? Had she taken a nap? Does she ask about me? Does she even notice I'm gone? I didn't think it was physically possible to love someone that much. But I did. I also wanted to be able to one day explain to her the tragic events in this pregnancy that led up to my leaving her at home while I went to the hospital for bedrest. I don't ever want her to think I abandoned her or that it was in any way easy for me.

"Missing my little girl, Abigail," I replied tipping my head down to hide the tears that were starting to trickle. I was hoping I wouldn't lose it in front of Caroline. "Let's start with that," I whispered.

"That's it! That's your song," she said with excitement. "Just write how you feel about being away from Abby."

I took a deep breath. This was going to be one hard song to write. "I'll try," I said.

Caroline put her hand on my shoulder and rubbed the top of my arm.

"I know this is upsetting, but I'd recommend starting with several minutes of free-writing, capturing all the thoughts that come to your mind without judgment. Then you can organize and re-structure it. Rhyming will come later. And don't worry about a melody just yet. I'll help with that. How about I check in with you tomorrow around 2:00 p.m.?"

"Okay," I said. "I'll start tonight and see what I come up with."

I went back to my room that afternoon and grabbed a snack out of the refrigerator and a fresh cup of water. I made a sign, using the white monitoring paper: "Napping, please do not disturb," and put it on my door. Jenny was working our pod that day. I filled her in on what I was doing.

"Sounds great, hun!" she said. "I'll make sure no one bugs ya, and I'll try not to bug ya myself. You have a few hours before your next monitoring." She glanced at the schedule at the nurses' station and then back at me. "By the way, tomorrow you have your biophysical ultrasound with Ashley, our technician."

"Oh good," I said and peered down at my belly. I couldn't wait to see what position the girls were in. No fighting in front of Ms. Ashley, I told them, and especially no fighting if Dr. Miller or Dr. Cooper walks into the room.

There was a knock on the door. Paul entered, carrying an assortment of junk food.

"I raided like four different vending machines looking for peanut butter M&Ms, I remembered you said they were your favorite."

"You are the best! Thank you." I grabbed the bag and tore it open, popping a few into my mouth.

"Want to watch a *Housewives* episode? They are having reruns all day on Bravo."

I laughed and nodded my head. "Of course, I'm always down for a good laugh with all their pomp."

Paul pulled up the lounge chair next to my bed and we chowed down on the rest of the snacks he'd brought. When the episode was over, he stood up, grabbed the wrappers on my bed and threw them away.

"Coffee date tomorrow?" he asked.

"Yes please, the usual nonfat, sugar-free latte."

"Got it," he said as he headed towards the door.

I grabbed a pen and some paper off my desk to begin working on my song. I scribbled down a few words. I was interrupted by a knock at the door. Dr. Cooper walked in. I found humor in the fact that everyone must have read the sign on my door, thought it didn't apply to them and proceeded into my room. I could have done without most of the daily interruptions including hospital staff checking my rooms inventory, the tech coming every few hours to check my vitals, and random volunteers with the bright red vests asking if I needed anything. But I always welcomed a visit from Dr. Cooper and Paul when he had food.

"Hey kiddo, I was in the area and thought I would check on you. Everything going okay?"

"Yeah, I'm working on a little musical project with the therapist intern."

"Oh, good for you. Staying busy and productive. I'll leave you to it then."

He started walking towards the door and saw the mound of junk food on my counter that had piled up from friends, family and Paul.

"I missed lunch and I have to run into surgery, would you mind if I grabbed a bar?"

"Are you kidding, I could feed an army, help yourself."

"Thanks. The kids and I are going to Costco this weekend, any requests?"

"Wine, lots of it," I smiled. "Just kidding. No, I'm good."

"Text if you change your mind," he said, opening the bar and taking a bite. He walked out the door and I picked up my pen and paper. I cleared all the junk—stress, worries and mundane nonsense out of my mind. And then I wrote. Just scribbles at first, random thoughts, and quickly, they came together to tell our story, the story of the day I left home. The day I left Abby.

While I've been gone, I've been thinking about you,
my sweet little Abby
Every day, all day long.
If I could choose, I would have had things go so differently
(of course)
Sometimes we get no say in things that happen in life.
I have to be strong and carry on.
I know this is temporary and it won't be this way forever.
Soon we will be together again, my Abigail.

As I finished the last line, I burst into tears. *Darn it. This was exactly why I didn't want someone walking in on me. Blubbering over my pen and paper, I would appear to be a hormonal mess. But geez was this hard.*

But then I thought: *What if journaling allowed me to move past that pain, even just a little? What if this whole writing thing proved to be cathartic, a type of therapy?* I didn't know, and hell, I could be completely wrong about this. But I figured I was just sitting there. I might as well give it a try.

I drank some water, took a deep breath and allowed my thoughts to transport me back to when I was pregnant with Abby. I was the picture-perfect example of a new mother-to-be. I had stayed within the recommended thirty-five pounds. I had lots of energy and was up and about with my big baby bump—teaching, working on the nursery, attending friends' weddings and fundraising galas and preparing for Abby's debut.

I can say it was easy in comparison to my hellish pregnancy with the twins. But, if you ask any mother, she'll tell you there's no such thing as an entirely easy pregnancy. I mean, you are growing a whole new person. There is *always* something unpleasant—morning sickness, hemorrhoids, or worse, a scare of some kind. Every mother shared the dreaded fear of not knowing if a healthy baby would be the result.

My pregnancy with Abby was no exception. I was already on edge after my first pregnancy had ended abruptly. I took a pregnancy test as soon as I thought there was the slightest possibility and was ecstatic to see we had conceived on our very first month of trying. Of course, I took four more tests just to be absolutely sure.

Though I was thrilled to be pregnant, I was also very cautious. Unlike the first time, I waited a few weeks before going to the doctor. I hoped that by the time I had my first ultrasound, we'd be able to hear a heartbeat. The last thing I wanted was to share the happy news with friends and family, only to have to tell them again that we had had another miscarriage. When I made it a little over a month after the positive test without any signs of spotting, I scheduled that first appointment.

At about nine weeks I went into see Dr. Cooper; he performed the ultrasound and confirmed that we had a sesame-seed sized baby with a heartbeat. Finally, for the first time since seeing the positive pregnancy test, I felt I could relax a little. The next big question was whether we would have a boy or a girl. For some reason, I felt like I was carrying a boy. At my next ultrasound, Dr. Melham, one of Dr. Cooper's partners, told me that, while it was still too early to paint the nursery, his best guess was that we were having a boy.

Two weeks later we went back for another ultrasound with Dr. Cooper.

"You're through the first trimester, so it's safe to share the news."

"I think I'm having a boy," I blurted.

"It's pretty hard to tell this early," Dr. Cooper admitted. "I'll venture a guess, but you really have to wait until the twenty-week ultrasound to draw any conclusions. For your twenty-week we will use the fancy schmancy machine upstairs that takes more powerful images."

I knew the machine he was talking about. When I had my miscarriage, I had been sent up to that office to have some imaging done to confirm the status of the pregnancy. Going back there would trigger all that old pain. I was worried about the things that might be revealed at the twenty-week scan, so of course I went. One, because I had to—doctor's orders—but two, we would be finding out the gender.

"So," he said, pausing while scanning my belly, "it looks to me like you're having a girl!"

"Really? Are you sure?" I was ecstatic. I had always wanted a little girl. Pink bows and ruffles, tutus and tiaras—I was in heaven.

"Positive," he said confidently.

I was once again excited and nervous. Ed and I decided that we needed to pick her name so we could start talking to her and calling her by name, instead of just "Baby Duffy." It would be nice for our family, too. They could get a jump on monogramming items for her, which is a popular thing in the South. We picked her middle name first—an easy decision—Micaela after my Ita, who had passed away two years before. For the first name, I spent countless hours looking at baby websites, weighing each consideration. Nope, too common. Ugh, too old-fashioned. Heck no, I had a former student with that name and I don't want it associated to our child. Eventually I compiled my short-list: Sophia, Olivia and Abigail.

I brought it up in conversation to my dad one day, and he confessed that he too had compiled a list of potential names for his future little princess.

"I love Abigail," he said sweetly. "I always have."

"Oh, wow!" I said. "That's incredible. Abigail is one of the names we are considering."

Such a sweet gesture from Grandpa; I thought it was meant to be. I ran it by Ed and he loved Abigail; he especially loved that we would call her Abby.

My twenty-four week ultrasound was a long process with a technician operating a large ultrasound machine in a dark room for what seemed like hours. She took a variety of measurements, but since she wasn't a doctor, she couldn't tell us anything. Of course, I would later encounter this issue again.

We anxiously waited until the next week when we were back in Dr. Cooper's office and he was looking over the report sent to him electronically from the technician. He went through every detail with us. "Her heart looks good. Lungs, liver and kidneys are all developing properly. Has the right number of fingers and toes," he joked. He continued to scan and then the room got very quiet. He hesitated, as if searching for the right words. I felt like I was waiting for the other shoe to drop. I braced myself for bad news I could sense was coming.

"There is one potential issue with the brain."

"What! Her brain?" I screeched.

"What kind of issue?" Ed asked quietly.

"The scan uncovered some cysts in the baby's brain, which are sometimes consistent with Trisomy 18. It's a condition that causes severe developmental delays due to an extra chromosome. But they didn't see any other indicators, just this one. It's something we will monitor."

There were no guarantees in medicine, especially in childbirth. You got what you got. This I knew. I also knew even back then that "something we will monitor" is doctor code for, "This is some serious shit that we are hoping will clear up on its own, but I can't tell you not to worry. Sorry."

"I'd like to send you to a perinatologist, Dr. Reiter, a specialist who will be able to do some more scans over the next few weeks. The cysts should resolve themselves on their own, in which case we'll have nothing to worry about." he said. His voice was serious, very un-Cooper like.

Dr. Bill basically regurgitated what Dr. Cooper said, but mentioned an even greater possibility of having a key indicator of Trisomy 18. Ed and I walked slowly out of the office. I saw a gift shop in the lobby. It was bright, meticulously organized and everything was objectively precious—the tiny onesies, the booties, the receiving blankets. I walked through the aisles of the store, brushing the softness with my fingers. Tears poured down my cheeks. If our baby was born with Trisomy 18, it would be a death sentence. A very small percentage of those babies lived past the age of five. And we'd be back where we started: baby-less.

We had plenty to worry about, think about and Google. I decided it was best for me not to do any research on the internet. I would leave that to Ed and instead try to focus on other things, like how my pregnancy had been up to that point, so healthy and strong. I had so much faith that everything would turn out okay. Things worked out the way they were meant to. They had to, right? Why would my body have allowed the pregnancy to progress that far if there was even the slightest chance of an issue?

If I was meant to have a baby with special needs, I would open my heart, embrace the baby and love him or her just as much. However, if I had a special needs baby, fell in love and then they died before the age of five, I knew I would lose my shit. Still, as much heartache and pain as I knew it would cause me, it would never make me chose to terminate my pregnancy. I would rather have that precious, but limited, time with my baby than no time at all. It was like that famous line from the Tennyson poem (which people commonly attribute to Shakespeare): "It is better to have loved and lost than never to have loved at all." I wholeheartedly agreed.

Ed continued to scour the internet for information on Trisomy 18. I could tell his in-depth research terrified him, but I wouldn't let myself go there. I was determined to stay intentionally uninformed and positive. "It's out of our hands," was my refrain whenever he broached the topic.

At around thirty-four weeks, at a routine ultrasound with Dr. Bill, our prayers were answered. The room was dark and quiet. He stared intently at the screen and wrinkled his nose, "It seems our issues have resolved themselves, as nature sometimes does." He pointed at the screen. "The cysts that were here are gone." Vanished just like that. We had spent almost every waking minute over the previous few weeks terrified that our baby would be born sick and we would only have him or her for a couple of years. Alleluia! Our baby was strong and healthy! I lid on that exam table and burst into tears. Ed squeezed me tight as tears rolled down my cheeks. The scanning gel ended up all over his sports coat.

Things were nice, quiet and uneventful for a while, but at thirty-eight weeks, Abby decided things were getting dull and so she was going to do some acrobatics. With her head faced downward, she did a somersault in my belly, landing in a breech position. Um okay, now what? I wondered. We discussed all the options with Dr. Cooper and decided that a C-section was the best and safest choice. Both because Abby was breech and did not seem to want to flip back—despite my endless attempts at acupuncture and various chiropractors—and she was (and always had been) measuring big in proportion to my petite frame. In my youth, I had always wanted a completely natural childbirth—a drug-free delivery in which I endured the pain—just as my grandmother had done and her mother before that. It had been so important to me before I was ever pregnant, but in that moment, when we were so close to giving birth, to meeting our little girl, I put my wants aside and picked the safest choice.

I woke up on the sweltering hot July morning with painful contractions. Thank goodness Ed hadn't left for work yet and he was available to drive me to the hospital. We arrived at the hospital at 10:00 a.m. and by 1:10 p.m. our Abigail was born at thirty-nine weeks on the dot, weighing a whopping nine pounds, two ounces. A big, strong, and healthy baby, she was busting out of the newborn size diapers the hospital provided.

"Whoa! Looks like we made the right decision," Dr. Cooper joked. "You could have labored for two days and ended up needing an emergency C-section anyway."

No joke there; I couldn't believe it.

From the moment I laid eyes on my baby girl, I was completely in love. I knew all moms were enamored with their first-born children, but I was over-the-top head-over-heels. She was, without a doubt, absolute perfection. Her nose was tiny and delicate, not squished at all since she had gotten to bypass the whole being squeezed out of the birth canal thing. Her head was rounded and she was completely bald (and would be until months later when her black ringlets would grow in). Her eyes were bright, star-gazing blue, perfectly matching her soft, rosy pink cheeks. Her little eyebrows were peach fuzz just faintly starting to grow in. Her feet were turned funny because of her breech position in utero, but I wasn't worried. She was as perfect as could be. I couldn't believe she was mine. In my arms, I felt like I was holding someone else's baby. I kept thinking that, at any moment, a nurse would come in and say, "Okay, Mrs. Duffy, time's up!" and I would have to give her back. I never wanted to put her down—not even to sleep. I stayed awake all night those first few nights, breathing in her scent of fresh air, ivory soap and lavender. I'd kiss her and her skin was so soft, like a piece of tissue paper. I would endlessly gaze at her, studying her every detail, kissing and stroking the top of her head. When I gazed into her eyes, I could see the universe in my tiny baby. I often wondered what did I do so right to deserve this little miracle. She's my firstborn—the one I will always have been most impacted by. Not just at birth, but every step of the way. She made me a mother first. It's because of her that I have a place in my heart overflowing with love. A love that is protecting and nurturing. Different from the love I have for Ed, this one welcomes cherished responsibility. A type of love that means that there is now someone who cannot go on without me—they need me in a way I had never been needed before, and that little life keeps on living because of me.

We were connected, her and I, bonded forever; I felt such overwhelming happiness. I knew it would carry me through any struggles we encountered. And it had. It had gotten me to where I was now.

My moments of reflection inspired my song lyrics. I picked the pen back up and wrote; and then I couldn't stop writing. Thoughts kept coming and words poured out on the page.

Soon we will all be together again
Between now and then, I want you—My Abigail—to know
that I love you
I miss you
I think of you every day
You are what my dreams are made of
I just can't wait to be back together again
While I'm away I'm thinking of you every day...

CHAPTER 15

EVERYDAY HEROES

For days, the creative spark remained, and I took full advantage of it in between my ultrasounds with Ashley, TV binge-watching with Paul, and daily visits from friends, family and Dr. Cooper. My outside visitors especially made for wonderful study breaks, and when we said our goodbyes, instead of getting sad, I channeled my emotions into my songwriting.

Since the morning I left
I could not forget your sweet face
The tears were running down all over my face
I had to go forward, and carry on

"You should use 'go on' since it rhymes with 'and carry on,' and we can place emphasis on the double r," Caroline suggested.

I found that I enjoyed my one-on-one time with Caroline way more than attending the group meetings. No one ever really participated. The moms that did show up just sat in their chairs, heads down, playing on their phones—as if the only reason they were there was because their doctors had made them go. My songwriting and talks with Caroline were a better use of time for me. So I stopped attending the group meetings altogether, but I did enjoy receiving updates from Caroline about the moms that had gone home and new ones that checked in.

We had settled into my routine after lunch one afternoon. The sun shined through the blinds, and Caroline sat by my bed playing country and jazz background music on her guitar.

I know it won't be this way forever
Soon we will all be together again

"Okay, so 'together again' can be your chorus," Caroline said. "This is amazing, Crystal, you are a natural songwriter."

We were cranking this song out together, but I took the compliment.

"Aww, thank you," I said as I blushed. "I've always loved writing. What is it they say that makes a great writer—writing about what you know. I guess I just needed some material, some intense feelings, to get me started."

The previous weeks had been such an emotional rollercoaster. One thing after another. It was around-the-clock worrying about the safety of my babies. I had had several sleepless nights in a row from long, stressful monitorings. There had been a different nurse each night, which definitely didn't help. One would find Katherine right away but then wouldn't be able to find Lauren, the wiggle worm, as I started calling her.

Baby girl, I love you, but you are stressing Mommy out, I told her. This can't be good for you either. And can I venture to guess that you might have been the one who tore the inner twin membrane? You either wanted to cuddle with Katie, or you just wanted to add more dramatic flair to your time in my womb. As if we need any more drama around here.

The more stressful things got, the more I threw myself into songwriting. Caroline and I explored several potential melodies. Too upbeat, too fast-paced, too out there. I finally chose one with a slow tempo and a soothing rhythm—perfect music for a melancholy, introspective song.

Dreaming of you while I'm away.
Being there to see your sweet face.
Setting off on adventures, on walks to the park.

"How about, 'When you look up at the *Goodnight Moon*, hope that you know that I'll be there soon. I miss you. Oh, Abby, I miss you.' We can change the tempo here for more effect."

"Oh my goodness, Caroline, you are a genius. I love that we incorporated Goodnight Moon, one of Abby's favorite books." I closed my notebook and looked up at Caroline. "Girl, you are something else. You seriously are my hero."

"Me?" she sounded surprised. "No, heroes risk their lives for our safety, like policeman and firefighters, or doctors and nurses who save lives."

"Well, not all heroes wear a uniform. Some heroes are people we encounter in our everyday life," I said.

She smiled and glanced down at her guitar. "I'm flattered," she said. "Giving someone the gift of music during a trying time in their life is incredible."

It was true. I hadn't wanted to admit that I was in therapy, but I suppose that was the purpose of music therapy; it didn't carry the stigma of traditional therapy and was more of a musical and creative process that simultaneously healed. Whatever it was, it worked really well for me. I needed the musical outlet to process my feelings, emotions and everything we had gone through. My song embodied everything about my experiences of motherhood and my incredible love and intense longing to be with my child. The song had a tremendous impact on me; it empowered me in so many ways, allowing me to process the pain and start moving past it. I had tried so hard throughout my pregnancy to not stress, to control my emotions, but I was only human. But I didn't want my time in the hospital to be tinged with despair. I didn't want to let myself sink into a hormonal depression. I didn't want to get so messed up from this experience that I would need traditional therapy when my babies were born. And that was just it; I didn't allow myself to think if my babies are born, but rather when they are born. I knew that when they were born, I'd be as busy as the President; I wouldn't make the time to heal or go to therapy. A mother always puts her children's needs above her own. Right or wrong, that was the reality, and I'd observed this countless times with my Ita. She was selfless and generous with her children and grandchildren. Even when her husband passed away and she was grieving his loss, she was able to pull strength from within and carry on. I was grateful both for that lesson and to have found comfort in songwriting, a beautiful pastime that allowed me to take care of myself. Something that might not have happened had I been home alone with Abby.

"Sorry to interrupt you, ladies," Jenny said as she strode into my room. "Crystal, I need to take you down to Ashley for your biophysical ultrasound."

"Okay, no problem. We're at a good stopping point." I turned toward Caroline. "See you tomorrow?"

"Yep, same time. I'll be here," Caroline said, and holding Jewel tightly, she skipped out of my room and down the hallway.

Jenny wheeled me down the hall and parked my wheelchair in the hallway. She knocked on the door of the exam room.

"I'll be right out," said a voice from the other side of the door.

Ashley, the ultrasound technician, opened the door. "Hi, honey! Sorry, just wrapping up some notes, but I'm ready for you." She looked down and rubbed my belly. "How are my precious baby girls today?" she said, peering down under my blouse.

I had met Ashley once, briefly, in the middle of the night. The night nurses were panicking after they had not been able to locate the babies or get a heartbeat. They needed to get a visual on the babies' location to be able to place the monitor on the correct location. What a rough night! I'd feared we had lost one or even both of the babies. We'd called Dr. Cooper on his cell phone and he arranged for an ultrasound tech to come to my room. In came Ashley like a guardian angel sent from heaven, with her magic ultrasound machine. In twenty seconds, she found Katie and Lauren, saving me from mass hysteria. Lauren had completely shifted positions. She had previously been on the right side of my stomach breech, but suddenly she was in the middle, lower, head facing down.

You little squirm bucket. You just want to be near Katie, I said to her. You are giving your mommy gray hairs, but that is the sweetest thing ever.

I often wondered why they didn't leave an ultrasound machine on standby in my room and just use that for every monitoring. I once asked Jenny and she told me, "Oh shug, those machines are super expensive, the hospital doesn't have that many of them floating around. Plus, as a nurse, performing an ultrasound is beyond the scope of our job. You need a technician or doctor to do it. Believe me though, it would make all of our lives easier if we could."

"If I live through this experience, I'd like to volunteer and advocate for that one day. More ultrasound machines readily available to antepartum patients," I said, making a mental note.

Ashley helped me onto the examining table.

"I can't wait to meet these two, Ash," I told her. "They are tenacious. I love it."

"I know they are, especially from what I can tell on the screen," she said. "I feel like I know their personalities already. Katie is gentle and sweet; Lauren is spunky and active. I wonder who takes after who?" And she winked.

"I have no idea," I said, sarcastically. I knew darn well that Lauren was every bit like her mama, whereas Katie was more Ed and Abby. "Do you have any plans for this long weekend?" I asked, changing the subject.

"Nope," she said, "I'll actually be working most of the weekend."

"What? No, you need a break from work—time to let loose and hang out with a fun guy." I playfully pushed her arm.

"Ha!" she snorted. "Not a chance. I'm almost forty, and I'm taking a break from men for a while." She paused and scratched her nose with her knuckle. "I had a painful break-up some years ago." Her expression turned somber.

Oh, shoot! Me and my big mouth. "I'm so sorry. I had no idea." I patted her arm again.

"No, that's okay."

She opened up and told me her back story. She was originally from Louisiana but had been living in California for school when she met her boyfriend. She dropped out of school and followed him to Texas where they dated for many years. They'd bought a house together. She thought that, after the major life purchase, an engagement would follow. He would always tell her, "Oh yeah, one day, but we have plenty of time." She kept waiting for "one day" to arrive. While looking through their kitchen junk drawer one afternoon, she came across a piece of paper that would change her life. She found a receipt for a two-night hotel stay at a fancy luxury hotel downtown. The dates were the exact same ones from a month before when she had gone home to Louisiana to visit her parents. Her boyfriend had lied and said he couldn't join her because he had to "work all weekend." She put all the details together and confronted him when he came home that evening. She discovered that the affair had been going on for months with a co-worker of his. "Screw you both, I'm done," she screamed at him while packing up her things. She moved out of the house, got her own place and went back to school. She'd always wanted to work in health care, a passion that stemmed from her own health problems. She shared that she had an auto-immune disease that worsened when she became sick.

"That's cool that you chose to become an ultrasound technician," I said, shifting positions on the chair.

"I've always loved babies, I wanted to find a job where I could help them but didn't involve direct patient interaction because of my illness. Plus, the salary is great."

"Nice!"

The conversation shifted back to weekend plans.

"How about you, missy? Is your family coming up?" she asked.

"Yes, Ed will bring Abby, and my sister-in-law, Bridget, is in town. Ed's cousin, Danny, who just moved to Houston, will be joining us too."

"Fun! Sounds like you will have a full room." She smiled, and then turned her attention to the ultrasound, moving the scanner all over my belly.

Memorial Day was coming up. In my previous life, I always planned a trip for us or hosted a barbecue. I thought back to the first summer after college when Ed and I moved in together. We had a teeny tiny studio apartment in Dupont, the hip part of Washington at the time. The oppressive heat reminded me of Texas summers—hot, sticky and humid, swarming with mosquitos. The weather gave me a bad case of hair flyaways at the top of my head. I was always so excited for Memorial Day, the holiday that kicked off summer. One year, we decided to throw a barbecue at our place. Ed and I were busy with preparations as the date drew near.

"Did you get enough burgers and hot dogs, Ed?" I asked him the night before. "So far everyone has RSVP'd "yes." Half of Washington is going to be on our rooftop."

"Yes, but I had to go to two different stores because—being a holiday weekend—Safeway was out of everything."

"Who runs out of buns?" I laughed.

Some of my best memories of our time in Washington were from that afternoon. A huge crowd of yuppies—mostly recent grads from Georgetown, GW and American—desperately trying to stay cool in our rooftop pool. There wasn't much room, but by the end of the night, we decided the more the merrier. We ordered pizza when the hot dogs ran out, and everyone was sharing beer. From the rooftop you could see Georgetown's main campus—Healy Hall tower. *That's where Ed and I met and our journey began,* I thought.

Ed and I had been dating a little over two years at that point; we were young and so carefree. I would never have imagined a mere seven years later—in a blink of an eye—I'd be spending the same national holiday with Ed and our family jammed in a frigging hospital room. No backyard BBQ or picnic, no pool party—just me as a science project.

I finished my ultrasound with Ashley, and Jenny wheeled me back to my room. I pulled out my phone and called Ed at work.

"So, want to come by to bring me dinner and drop off some clean clothes?" I knew the answer, but I still wanted to ask nicely. "You know, I was just thinking about that first summer we spent in Dupont. Remember the rooftop pool party?"

"Ahh, yes. That seems like so long ago."

"Yeah, those days are long gone."

Ed chuckled. "Well, don't be so sure," he said.

I sighed. "I really don't see how we are going to do much of anything this year, seeing how I have to ask permission to even get wheeled down the hall."

"I may not be able to take you to a fun, rooftop party or the beach, but I promise I'll make this Memorial Day special for you," Ed said. "Abby and I have a little something planned."

On Memorial Day, my family arrived one-by-one, each carrying what seemed like more stuff than usual. Bridget pushed Abby in the stroller. Danny had some grocery bags containing what I could only imagine was some snacks for us—which was perfect because I was starving. Ed came in last, holding our large white laundry basket from our home. What in the world?

"So, we decided since we couldn't take you to a party, we were going to bring the party to you!" Ed said. He smiled as he revealed his surprise. He'd stuffed the basket with plates, napkins, plastic cutlery and cups. There were condiments and more chips and salsa. Then he pulled out one last thing from the laundry basket.

"Oh my goodness! You snuck in a grill?" I exclaimed.

It was a decent-sized grill from William Sonoma that sat perfectly on our counter at home—a wedding present from Uncle Bob. We had spent countless hours together grilling up delicious meals.

"That's so incredibly sweet, honey," I said as I threw my arms around his neck and planted a kiss on his cheek. "But…"

"But what?" he said.

"What if the nurses find out?"

"Don't worry. If someone comes by, we can just offer them a delicious grilled burger or hot dog in exchange for their conspiring silence."

"I can't believe you did this, Ed," I told him. "You are my hero."

DEEPENING TENSIONS

The Memorial Day party had been fun, we grilled all the burgers and hots dogs and had some nurses and even the chaplain on duty come by and hang out with us. Weekends were usually a slow time at the hospital since the doctors weren't around, but we did have a resident—a young female doctor from Dr. Cooper's office—come by in the evening to check on me and join in our hospital room party. Tuesday, after the holiday, things went back to usual at the hospital. This week marked week twenty-seven.

"Well, look at this," Jenny said as she rubbed my stomach with scanning gel. "What cute little hearts! Did Ashley draw those?" There were two little black hearts drawn in with a black sharpie on my belly. They looked like tattoos.

I nodded. "Yeah, she drew them at my ultrasound Friday morning because she wanted to find a way to make twin-tracking easier," I said. "I was telling her about how rough the night monitorings have been. The girls keep moving so much; it's been hard to track them down, and more importantly, keep them on track for a long enough stretch for a good report."

It had been all Ashley's idea. She was so thoughtful, always trying to help others. In this case, her nurse friends. She was so excited about the belly hearts.

"Just watch," I said, "the girls will interfere with Ashley's good intention of trying to help you out. I bet by tonight they'll be in completely different locations."

Jenny laughed. "Probably, but for right now, it is very much appreciated."

As time wore on, I felt my initial optimism and positive attitude fading. More emotional and traumatic stress just piled and piled on top of older worries and stress from the recent months. When would it stop? Or the very least just stay the course? Each monitoring brought us closer to our delivery day. And, while I knew the babies were okay, a part of me feared something awful would still happen. But how could it? Really, what else could possibly go wrong? I remembered Dr. Cooper's words the day he told me I was going inpatient. "Never," he'd said, "in my thirty years of practicing medicine have I ever seen a pregnancy like this one."

The rest of that week flew by with continued visits from Dr. Cooper, Dr. Miller, family and friends. That next Monday, June 2, my Aunt Michelle checked into the hospital and gave birth via C-section to her third son, my youngest cousin, Andrew. Having her and newborn Andrew there in the hospital—in the room right next to mine per my request— reminded me of home. Her four-day hospital stay was filled with non-stop visits from family, home cooked meals delivered to our room, late night talks and endless cuddling with eight-and-half-pound baby Andrew. I laid him across my swollen belly. "Meet your cousin, Katie and Lauren," I said as they kicked me fiercely from the inside. They were instant playmates. The day Michelle and Andrew got discharged was painful. My happy distraction was gone and my thoughts were once again filled with fear and terror. I reflected on everything.

We had come so far; we had survived the deadly TTTS, the laser ablation surgery, the septostomy and several weeks in the hospital with constant monitoring. I was close to thirty weeks. Before the surgery, we didn't even know if I would make it this long; thirty weeks was a major milestone. Every day in the hospital was a huge accomplishment and would mean less time for the twins in the NICU. They were beyond the point of being micro preemie (a baby weighing less than a pound) which was reassuring if something happened and we had to deliver. But then why couldn't I relax more?

My mind had been wrapped up in life as an inpatient. I had lost track of the days. We were a couple of weeks into June already. My wedding anniversary on the twelfth was fast approaching. I had been a June bride. I was twenty-five then—beautiful, not a wrinkle on my face, not a gray hair on my head nor a scar on my body. I was thin—a solid size two. Ha! Good luck to me losing all the baby weight again. My wedding ring sparkled on my finger, just as it had on that happy day. My wedding is a day I will always remember, I thought, as I rotated my ring around my finger.

Jenny had just finished tracking the girls on the monitor and was fastening the elastic belt in place over my belly. She caught a glimpse of my ring, which sparkled in the sunlight coming through my window. "Your ring is beautiful, honey."

"Thank you," I said. "My anniversary is coming up this week."

"Is it really? How many years?"

"Four. Hard to believe. They've flown by." I paused. A lot had happened since that day. "We probably won't even celebrate this year," I sighed.

"Oh no, are you kidding me? Your husband is so romantic, I'm sure he's got something special planned," Jenny said, tapping my shoulder.

"I'm not really in the mood to celebrate," I said. "I know this sounds terrible, but sometimes I just think how different things would be if we had waited to have our second child. Maybe, just maybe, things would have gone differently." I began to tear up. I looked down at my tummy and rubbed it. I'm sorry, girls, I told them silently. I don't mean that—it's just the stress and worries are getting to me. I'm glad I didn't wait. I want you two to be ours.

"Oh, sweetie, don't say that," Jenny said. "I know it's so hard being stuck in here, away from your daughter, but don't lose sight of the amazing thing you have going on in there." She bent down and rubbed my belly. "I would have given anything to have been pregnant with twins. Shoot! Any second child as long as he or she were healthy." She dropped her eyes and stopped talking.

"Oh, I'm so sorry, Jenny. I didn't know." I said as I reached for her arm.

Jenny was gorgeous—that blonde curly hair, blue eyes and a great body—but there was an undeniably sad look in her eyes. Sometimes she would get very quiet and stare off into space. I had always wanted to know her backstory, but didn't want to pry.

"It's okay, I've had a while to come to terms with it," she confessed. And then, she shared her story.

It started with a physical attraction to an Elvis impersonator at a traveling show in Houston. It was an unofficial nurse night out. Jenny and her co-workers had gone to a few bars; they had been drinking heavily, pounding down gin and tonics and martinis. It wasn't hard to imagine the scene—Jenny as a party girl. During a cigarette break outside the bar, she met Roberto, the handsome Latino charmer who had just walked off the stage. Jenny had always been a huge Elvis fan. She had been raised listening to all his tunes, and here she had bumped into someone who shared her love for his music. This guy was tall, dark and handsome with a Spanish accent—a walking cliché. He reeled her in with his good looks, charm and suaveness.

Two months later, they were wed at a small chapel in Vegas. Wedding officiant—Elvis, of course. Five months later she gave birth to their daughter.

"How old is your baby?" I leaned in closer.

"Presley is five, starting kindergarten this fall. I can't believe it."

"Presley? Of course," I interrupted. "I love it!"

She paused and then blurted, "Roberto and I split up."

Dammit! I thought. I was really rooting for a happy ending.

"Oh, Jenny, I'm so sorry." I handed her a tissue. "What happened?"

"We had been married about three years when we broached the topic of getting pregnant again. We had both discussed having more children, and well, I wasn't getting any younger. The thing that had kept us from trying sooner was that Presley was a handful. She had bad colic and reflux and would cry all night. It only worsened my postpartum depression. With the support and love from family and friends, I sought medical attention and improved. We tried getting pregnant for over a year and a half. I managed to get pregnant once, but suffered an early miscarriage. I didn't take it well, and my depression returned. Roberto and I started to grow apart—all the trying and failing was wearing on our relationship. The more we wanted it and the harder we tried, the more we failed. At long last, I was pregnant when I was just shy of thirty-seven. I ignored all the warnings—you know the ones about trying to conceive after thirty-five—and the high risk of having a child with medical problems or disabilities. I wasn't going to worry about something out of my control that hadn't even happened yet."

This sounded familiar. I hear ya, girl.

"At twenty weeks, during our big ultrasound scan, we learned we were having a boy. We also found out our boy had Down syndrome. We were crushed. Devastated. Heartbroken. This is it, I thought, this is my last chance to be a mother of two. I wasn't going to get another opportunity. I had struggled so much just getting pregnant this time around, despite having conceived Presley so easily. I was faced with the most difficult decision of my life. Do we continue this pregnancy knowing we will bring a little boy into the world with severe, life-long health problems, or do we terminate the pregnancy, save him from a life of grief and save ourselves from more heartache?"

I was sitting on the edge of my seat as I waited for Jenny to continue, even though I already knew how her story would end.

"As a nurse, I've seen it all. I knew about Down syndrome and the lifetime of health issues. Would he be able to talk? Would he learn to read and write? Was I prepared to deal with this if he couldn't? No matter how many doctor's appointments or therapy sessions we went to, nothing was ever going to change. Our boy would never be cured, and knowing this, we as his parents would have decided to proceed nonetheless. It was clear to me what we needed to do. My medical experience and my instincts prompted me to terminate the pregnancy, spare him a life of misery and spare ourselves and Presley the pain. But my heart broke—the part of me that wanted so badly to keep him, the part of me that thought I would later regret my decision. How would I live with myself?

"Roberto said to me over and over that ending his life wasn't the right thing to do. It was easy for him to say he didn't really know what this diagnosis meant for our family. But ultimately, he grew tired of the fight and said I should do what I thought was best for our family. In the end, I decided to terminate the pregnancy short of twenty-one weeks before any chance of viability.

"Roberto and I grieved and coped in our own ways, but not in ways that brought us together, ones that drew us apart. He went back to work doing his Elvis gigs. He traveled a lot. My depression returned; I was vulnerable because I had been off medication for the baby. I was so deeply lost in my depression that I wasn't able to repair myself, let alone my marriage. I lost the baby. I lost love and support from my family, and many of my friends—the ones that were passionate pro-life—stopped speaking to me altogether. And then I lost my husband."

She paused and took a breath.

"We agreed to an amicable divorce. We wanted to continue to co-parent Presley as best we could and keep open communication."

Jenny stopped and wiped her tears with a tissue. She perked up and continued.

"That was two years ago. I'm much better now. Happier, that's for sure. I'm dating someone. He's nothing like Roberto, and so far, it's going great. I'm having a lot of fun with it."

Just when I thought she had finished pouring out her heart to me she added one last thing.

"I never thought that my life would go quite this way. I used to stay up at night thinking of all the 'what ifs.' I realized I needed to accept that things happened a certain way for a reason. I wasn't meant to be a mother of two and that's okay. I absolutely adore my little girl, and I'm fine with the way things worked out."

She took a deep breath and exhaled with a sigh.

"Oh, wow," she said. "I hope I didn't overshare and make you uncomfortable. I'm sorry. I'm usually very professional with my patients. It's just, we've become so close and…"

"No, not at all, Jenny." I interrupted. "I'm so glad you did. You've been through so much. And you did what was right for you and your family. I'm really proud of you; what you did took tremendous courage."

I leaned over my bed and hugged her. She cried into my chest as I held her close. She had been there for me for weeks and had given me whatever I needed every single time I needed it. I was happy I could do something for her. Very few people really open up and share their hearts with you. Sometimes it takes years of friendship to reach that level of intimacy. Other friendships never come anywhere close.

"All that talking, and I didn't even notice you're done," Jenny said glancing at the monitor report by the machine. She dried the corner of her eyes with a tissue.

"Let's get these ribbons off and you can rest for the night," she said and unplugged me. She rolled up the elastic bands, placing them back in the drawer. And then she tidied up my room and said, "Goodnight, sugar." The mothering and nurturing from my nurses soothed me. As they tucked me into bed, it was as if they were recharging me like the battery of an iPhone. My babies and I were alone for the night, and my mind was running like crazy.

There I sat in the hospital, desperately trying to keep my babies alive, hoping and praying they would be born healthy. But I'd love them unconditionally no matter what the outcome. I'd become close with Jenny—my main caregiver—who was helping me survive the whole ordeal, and she had just confided in me that she chose to terminate her own pregnancy because of a difficult diagnosis.

In my pre-kid days, I had judged people who'd made that choice. Why would they end an innocent life? I didn't know shit about high-risk pregnancies and complications. But I did now, and I knew Jenny. After hearing her perspective, her issues and her life story, it all made sense. She wanted to stay healthy; she didn't want to fall back into depression.

She wanted to be strong for her daughter. And she knew deep down that she couldn't handle the pressure, stress, and immense pain that accompanied being a parent to a special needs child. And that's okay. She had the courage to make a painful decision. How could I ever judge anyone's difficult decisions again?

My thoughts turned to my babies. We had hoped and prayed for them to heal from the twin to twin disease, and they had. But so much was still unknown. They could be born at any moment, or they could die at any moment. They could be healthy or have serious birth defects.

I heard a tap on the door. Jenny popped her head in the doorway. "What day is your anniversary again, sugar?"

"Thursday, the twelfth."

"Oh, okay. I was just wondering if I was working that day, and it just so happens that I am." She smiled and left the room.

CHAPTER 17

FOR BETTER OR WORSE

I'd kept busy the days leading up to our anniversary—my regular round-the-clock monitorings, biophysical ultrasounds with Ashley and visits from my friends, my mom and dad and, of course, Abby. I even saw my sister Melissa. She'd been in Austin working during much of my pregnancy—it was nice to catch up with her too. I saw Caroline almost every day. On the days we didn't work on music, we just talked. She would keep me company, and if I was lucky, she would serenade me. She knew old rock classics like the Beatles and contemporary music like Justin Bieber. One time my dad and Abby arrived just as Caroline was leaving, but she stayed and played songs for us including Abby's request, "Elmo's Song" from Sesame Street. Abby's face lit up and she sang along with glee.

"Together Again" was finished and recorded. Caroline and I had spent over two hours recording and re-recording to get just the right take. She would play the melody on her guitar, and I was lead vocal with Caroline singing my backup. We used a sophisticated recording program through her laptop that would help edit the song. But, even with the advanced editing features, if I accidentally coughed or took a breath or paused for too long, we would have to re-do the whole thing. Now I knew how Adele felt. It didn't help that my hospital room was always as busy as Grand Central Station during Christmas time— nurses, doctors, technicians, volunteers, hospital chaplains—it was getting to the point where we couldn't go five minutes without someone barging in on us. We put a sign on the door that said, "Do Not Disturb," but every individual in the hospital seemed to think they were exempt from that sign—that somehow their task or job triumphed over anything that I had going on inside. It was an annoyance that I soon grew tired of.

I wished I had some semblance of privacy and space. A place where I could lock the door for a few minutes. Not even the bathroom had a lock in case there was a medical emergency. I was also nowhere near a professional singer, but I still wanted to capture this song just right. Leave it to me to continue to be a perfectionist even while in the hospital, a trait of mine I know bugged Ed. "Perfect is the enemy of good," he'd tell me. "Enemy or not, I still want it," I'd reply.

But "Together Again" was finally done!

I asked Caroline one afternoon, "Caroline, would you mind coming in and helping me perform the song live for Abby? I know she'd love that."

"Aww of course," she replied. "Just let me know when, and I'll be sure to bring Jewel."

"You mean sometimes you leave Jewel at home, all alone?" I teased.

Caroline laughed. "Jewel and I are pretty much attached at the hip. She's my baby."

"Wait until you have your own baby, then Jewel will be sleeping in the office chair," I giggled.

"No way," she said, shaking her head.

"I'm telling ya, girl. Life changes when there are little ones around."

Completing my song gave me such a rush of giddy excitement. My song was definitely another one of my babies. I had poured my heart and soul into making it and thought about it every time I wasn't directly thinking about Abby, Katie or Lauren. It enveloped every ounce of emotion I'd been experiencing—all the pain, sorrow and heartbreak, but it had all come together so beautifully. It had become so much more than just a piece of music, and I couldn't wait to share it with Abby.

My dad brought Abby to the hospital the next morning, the day of my anniversary. Abby was clutching a lollipop and held hands with her Elmo doll. She was ecstatic to see Mama, and I felt the same way about seeing her. They arrived as I was mid-monitor, belly exposed and wrapped tightly with the elastic bands, and she ran to the bedside, dropping both her doll and candy. She climbed up the side of the bed, and I leaned forward to kiss her head. And then I picked up my phone and quickly texted Caroline.

Our big performance debut, are you free now?

Yes, I'll be right down.

I was so excited for this moment, a tad nervous too. The sight of Caroline eased my nerves because I knew we would be doing this together. We chatted, laughed and giggled together while I finished up the time on the monitor.

Abby ran around the room, twirling her smock dress, eating up all the attention she was getting.

"Miss Abby." Caroline bent down to toddler height. "What song would you like me to play for you? What about 'Twinkle, Twinkle, Little Star?'"

"Aww, that would be great," my dad said, smiling at Abby.

"Elmo!" Abby exclaimed.

"Abby how about 'Twinkle, Twinkle' and then 'Elmo.' And say please," I said.

"Okay Mama, peez," she said cutely.

As Caroline played her songs, I started to tear up.

La, la, la, la Elmo's world
Elmo loves his goldfish, his crayons too
That's Elmo's world.

Man, you would think she just finished playing "Amazing Grace" at a soldier's funeral from all the emotion she evoked in me. How in the world was I going to keep a dry eye while singing my own song? As Caroline was finishing up "Elmo's Song," Jenny walked in to take me off the monitor.

"Jenny," I said, "I'm about to perform my song to Abby, if you want to stay and listen."

"I'd love to, sugar. I've been so curious as to what you and Miss Caroline have been up to in here these past couple of weeks."

There was a quick knock on the door.

Dr. Cooper came in, "Hey Crystal, looks like you have a room full of visitors. I can come back later."

"No, please stay Dr. Cooper, I'm about to perform my song that I wrote for Abby."

He smiled and stepped into the room next to Jenny.

I now had a full-on audience. My dad was videotaping it to show Ed and Gigi who were at work. Caroline handed me a sheet of paper. She'd typed up the lyrics to "Together Again."

"I got this, girl," I said, and smiled, pushing the sheet away.

"I know you do," she said, smiling back. "One, two, three..."

She strummed a note on Jewel, which was my cue to start. The words fell out of my mouth and filled the room, just as we had practiced. The first few verses were so familiar to me. I'd sung them so many times. By the time the chorus came around my voice really filled the room. I kept my eyes on Abby's face. She listened quietly, so taken by the performance, her little eyes full of excitement. The melody and instrumental-only part came, and I was grateful for a chance to catch my breath and look around at the smiles on Jenny and my dad's faces.

I then repeated the chorus. We were nearing the end—the start of the bridge, my special verse that had been made to a slightly different tempo.

Dreaming of you while I'm away,
being there to see your sweet face,
setting off on adventures, on walks to the park,
when you look up at the good night moon,
hope that you know that I'll be there soon,
I miss you, Oh Abby I miss you.

I finished the stanza and Abby yelled, "Mama," and ran over to my bed, lifting her arms above her head for me to pick her up. Jenny swooped in and lifted her onto the bed for me. I was hugging her so tightly that I forgot about finishing my song. I began to cry. Luckily, Caroline knew the lyrics by heart and brought the song to a close for me as I clutched Abby, stroking her hair and breathing her in.

Later that same day I started working on a song for Katie and Lauren, inspired by, Wherever You Are, My Love Will Find You, a children's book by an author named Nancy Tillman that I had read to Abby countless times. I loved it, not only for the beautiful unique illustrations, but also because the author writes about motherhood with a passion I found inspiring. The song's tempo was more fast-paced than the one I had written for Abby. Even though things were still precarious, I knew it had to be that way, or I wouldn't be able to write it. I would start to bawl if the beat was slow and introspective. Even so, it was incredibly difficult to write—especially since I still didn't know the outcome of my pregnancy. I wanted the babies delivered safely to my arms more than ever. We were approaching the gestation period in which they would be in more danger in my womb than outside in the NICU, but Dr. Cooper, as he mentioned earlier on his visit, still thought it was too early to do a voluntary C-section. The preemie risks were still super high. Any number of things could still happen.

My worries transcended themselves into song lyrics.

So many times, when I thought of you, I worried for your life
that you'd be okay.
I'd pray that you'd come to me safely.
I always remained strong in my faith, and knew that the
good Lord would deliver you,
Into my arms, sweet babies of mine. It was only just a
matter of time.
I'm singing this to you now, and I'll sing it again when you
are in my arms.
There has never been anyone just like you. You are
amazing, unique and beautiful too.
I love you my darlings and I'll always be with you.

I hope you girls like your song Mommy wrote for you, I told them after I'd finished my first draft and read it aloud to them. In response, I felt a flutter of kicks inside me. I took that as a "yes."

Later that same day, as the sun set on the evening of my wedding anniversary, the fading light filtered through my blinds. It was quiet and calm in my room, the way it usually was during a shift change. The day nurse was briefing the night nurse, who had just arrived for the evening. The doctors had gone home; only the on-call residents remained. Most visitors had cleared the floor. The dinner rush was over—all the meals had been delivered and the trays cleared; I hadn't eaten since I was waiting on Ed to bring us outside food.

I sat on my bed, legs crossed, waiting for Ed. I had showered and blow-dried my hair with a slight curl at the bottom—just the way he liked it. I had applied mascara, lipstick and blush to my pale cheeks after my monitoring. Ed would be arriving soon and we would be "celebrating" our anniversary. Just a chill night in my good ol' hospital room with take-out. As I waited, my thoughts drifted back to that happy, joyous June afternoon on which we, college sweethearts, had exchanged vows and pledged to always love and be there for one another. I could still picture myself saying the words aloud.

"I take, you, Edward, to be my lawfully wedded husband, to have and to hold, from this day forward, for better or worse, for richer or poorer, in sickness and in health, until death do us part." We were definitely in the midst of our "or worse" part. Who knew that it would come so soon after being married? I expected the worst part to be later in life during the years of declining health, not during what I thought was the prime of my life.

There was a faint knock on the door. Ed peeked in. "Sorry I'm a little late," he said. "I was helping out with something." He smiled.

He was indeed about half an hour late. I assumed it had been for work. I rolled my eyes, a little annoyed. Not only was he late, but he had also showed up empty-handed. Oh man, no flowers or even a card. Some anniversary celebration this would be. I was disappointed, almost at the verge of tears, when he interrupted my thoughts.

"Crys, you look beautiful," he said. Ha right, I thought, I look just like Shamu does before a big show at SeaWorld.

"And how are my little peanuts doing?" he asked, putting his face next to my belly, giving it a pat and a gentle kiss. "I've missed my girls, you three—well, four—have been on my mind all day." Before I could say anything, he extended his arm, offering me his hand.

"Crys, come with me. I have something to show you."

What in the world? He helped me off the bed and out the door. His assistance reminded me of a sweet grandson helping his eighty-five-year-old grandma walk. There was a wheelchair parked outside my room with two balloons tied to either side that said "Happy Anniversary." Laying across the seat of the chair were two big bouquets of red roses.

"Oh, they are gorgeous." I said cheerfully.

I picked up the roses and inhaled their lovely aroma. "Thank you, Ed."

"Here, get into your chariot," he said, standing behind the wheelchair.

"Wait, what? Where are we going?" I asked as I sat down.

He shrugged his shoulders as if he didn't know and smiled silently.

Baby girls, I'm not sure where Daddy is taking me, I told the twins. I think all three of us hope it involves food!

He pushed me down a familiar route past the other pods, other nurses' stations, and the vending machine to the end of the hallway. We stopped in front of the conference room where we held our antepartum group meetings.

"Why are we here?"

He put the wheelchair on break-mode, helped me out, then led me through the door. I hardly recognized the conference room. The usual bright, fluorescent lights were dim and white, glittery stars made from cardstock tied onto ribbon hung from the ceiling. A starched white, linen tablecloth was draped over the long conference table. All but two of the table's chairs had been pushed aside. Two illuminated candles were surrounded by a pair of flower arrangements—white and pink roses with a pink satin bow tied around the small glass vase. Red and pink rose petals had been scattered across the tablecloth. Two place settings were positioned next to each other, and beneath the covers on the fine, white china, there was something that smelled delicious. There were goodies on either side of the entrees—a fruit platter with delicious mangos, pineapple, strawberries and kiwi; chocolate chip cookies and little pink cupcakes with sprinkles on them. It was a feast featuring all of my favorite things.

A banner with the word "love" written on it was draped across the back wall. Silver and white balloons filled each corner of the room. There was a small table featuring three pictures I recognized from our living room. One photo framed Ed and me standing in front of Rockefeller Center a couple of months after we had started dating. One captured us on our wedding day, smiling in our get-away car. And the third was our most recent family picture—Ed, Abby and me sitting together on a park bench last winter. Music played softly in the background, a remix of "Love Story," another one of my favorites.

I was completely blown away. It was the most elegant, romantic room I had ever seen. And it had been done for me. My eyes brimmed with tears. I turned to Ed. "Babe, did you do all this?"

He shook his head. "No, Jenny. It was all her idea. She recruited Susan, Paul, Caroline, Ashley and me to help. She stayed way after her shift finishing up the last-minute touches."

Tears streaked my cheeks. I heard the clip-clop of footsteps behind me. I turned around to see the whole bunch of them standing in the doorway. I slowly waddled over to them.

I reached for Jenny and wrapped my arms around her. "How can I ever thank you for this? It's absolutely beautiful," I whispered into her ear.

She beamed. "I was happy to do it, honey."

"Y'all," I said looking at the five of them, "this seriously is the nicest, most thoughtful thing anyone has ever done for me."

Susan touched my shoulder. "You are the sweetest, strongest, most positive patient, and you have touched us with your spirit and your journey."

"We wanted to do something special for you," Caroline chimed in.

"Now, you will always remember your fourth anniversary—the one you spent here with us," said Ashley as she hugged me.

"This is so incredible. I will treasure this memory always. Thank you for this amazing gift." We embraced in a group hug.

"Please don't let us keep you from your evening," Paul said as he wiped a tear from his cheek.

"You have the room all night," Susan said. It felt like my mom telling me I had no curfew. I laughed.

"Ed picked up something good for you. It smells delicious," Ashley said.

"Enjoy, shug. You deserve it," Jenny said as they walked out and closed the door behind them.

I sat down, mopping my tears. My runny mascara stained my hands. "I can't believe this. It's so incredibly sweet. How lucky am I?"

"I know." Ed agreed. "Jenny told me on Monday that she wanted to plan something, and I was to keep the secret and go along with it." He took the lid off of our dinner. "I'm glad you were surprised," he said and then added, "Oh, and I picked up Mark's."

"Mark's. Wow," I shouted. "My favorite!" I sounded like a toddler.

We had eaten at Houstonian favorite Mark's restaurant, an old church converted into an elegant restaurant, the night we got engaged. We had many wonderful memories of dining there.

After we finished eating and listening to the fabulous playlist of classic love songs Caroline had compiled for us, we sat and talked for a long time. We talked about our worries and concerns for the twins' safety, memories we had of Abby, of our time living in DC before we were parents, our carefree college days. But mainly, we spoke of the wonderful things the future had in store of us when we got through this rough bit we were in.

The Beatles song, "In My Life" started to play. Ed pushed his chair back, stood up and offered me his hand. "Dance with me."

"Here?" I laughed.

"Why not? We have this incredible romantic room all to ourselves."

We had danced to this song at our wedding. I closed my eyes and I was there, reliving it all again.

The music from the band had filled the grand 1913 historic ballroom, which was resplendent with crystal chandeliers, heroic murals and thirty-five foot ceilings. There was laughter and giddy conversation coming from the outside wraparound terrace. The waiters filled champagne flutes as Ed and I joined our guests on the dance floor as a newlywed couple. Bright lights forming our initials "C" and "E" on the dance floor shined down upon us. He held me close and then spun me out and twirled me, just as we had practiced in our dance classes weeks before. "Mrs. Duffy," Ed whispered in my ear, "you've made me the happiest guy in the world by being my wife."

I blushed and smiled. "We are officially a family, you and I." I paused to look around at our family and friends and saw our little cousins running around the dance floor. "And someday our family will grow again. It's what I've always dreamed of."

He hugged me tightly. "Me too." And then he kissed me.

I was as happy in that moment as I had been then—I was building a family with this special man who had been there for me during the time I most needed him to be. For better or for worse, in sickness and in health. Our vows took on new meaning. Back then, I had no idea what we would be going through four years and a blink later. Even with the high-risk pregnancy—I wouldn't have it any other way.

We danced slowly, although pretty far apart given the size of my stomach, until the music stopped. I was so swept away in his arms; I almost forgot we were in the hospital.

BLESSINGWAY

"So how was dinner?" Paul asked over Friday morning coffee the next day. "It reminds me of an episode of Grey's Anatomy. Like your own little romantic retreat for the night." He smiled and took a sip of coffee.

"Delicious, but I was blown away by the whole thing."

"Oh, I know, right? The room was decorated so cute," Paul agreed.

"I wish I could stay and visit longer." Paul said looking down at his phone. "But I have a new patient checking into our unit. You remember how that goes," Paul said.

"Indeed, it feels like I've been here for months instead of just weeks."

Some girlfriends were scheduled to visit me later that day. My friends Sarah, Nicky and Sloane brought me lunch; we were indulging on taquitos and chips and queso. I would've killed for a margarita on the rocks with salt along the rim.

"So, everything is set and ready to go for your blessingway next week." Sarah said. "I just double-checked the responses—we have eight RSVPs, plus your mom, mother-in-law, Melissa and Abby. Thirteen total including you. It's this Tuesday at 4:00 p.m. We're planning on getting here half an hour before or so to set up."

I had already had a baby sprinkle for the twins. Normally, for second child you wouldn't do another traditional baby shower, but since we were having twins I thought it would be very helpful to stock up on two of everything. I wanted to do something different instead of a baby shower. My friend Sloane had something called a blessingway earlier that year for her second daughter, Lily—which I wasn't able to go to because I was already on bedrest at the beginning of my pregnancy— and I had fallen in love with the idea. A blessingway, or mother blessing, was an old Navajo ceremony in which family and friends celebrate the mother's passage into motherhood. Rather than bringing gifts for the baby, this special gathering is all about nurturing the mother-to-be and celebrating the joys of motherhood. Each woman in attendance is encouraged to share her own birth experiences and provide advice, wisdom and prayers for the mother-to-be.

I had invited Jenny, Susan, Caroline, Ashley and Paul as well as some of my other nurses to my celebration. My mom and my sister, Melissa, arrived at my room first with Abby. My mother-in-law, Kathy, was there too. She had flown in from California for the occasion. I had told her it wasn't necessary, but she wanted to be there. Together, we all loaded into an elevator and headed up to the tenth floor of the hospital to the event room. The room was bright and colorful with huge windows that overlooked the zoo. The energy felt warm and inviting without all the hustle and bustle of the labor and delivery floors. The walls were painted in shades of orange, green, yellow and purple, and the air was full of the smell of the freshly baked chocolate chip cookies waiting in the kitchen for kids and guests. The room held a new, shiny playground with several big pieces of equipment and lots of toys. There was a slide and a see-saw, a jungle gym and a rock wall. The only thing missing from this dream playroom were children. The space needed laughter and noise to bring it to life. But most of the patients on the floor were extremely ill children who couldn't get out of bed, or post-op patients who weren't here long enough to experience the room's magical essence. Something so beautiful that the mere sight of it made me want to burst into tears thinking about the sick children that couldn't play there. That and the whole hormones thing—always the hormones thing. I closed my eyes, took a deep breath and wiped a tear from my cheek.

"All right," I said as I motioned to Melissa to help me out of the wheelchair. "Shall we?"

As I carefully stepped out of the wheelchair, I turned and saw Abby. My precious little Abby was wearing a bright-colored floral sundress and had her hair in pigtails. Her little white sandals were decorated with flowers and jewels that sparkled when she walked. I remembered very clearly the day that we bought them. I had taken her to the mall to buy a couple of things for our upcoming trip to San Antonio: a pink rash guard swimsuit, white sun hat, polka dot Minnie sunglasses—she was going to be the most stylish toddler on the Sesame Street splash pad at SeaWorld. We were just missing shoes. I was looking for a pair of water shoes, the kind she could wear on the splash pad so she wouldn't burn her little feet, but I wasn't having any luck. And that's when she found those little jeweled, sparkly ones.

"Mama, can we buy these?" she asked, picking up her preferred pair.

"Baby girl, you need water shoes," I'd said. "These will get ruined in the water."

"Mama—let's buy two," she replied, "these and the water shoes… Then I'll be so happy." Her bright blue eyes lit up.

How in the world could I say no? The girl loved her shoes and she did have a great sense of style—which she obviously inherited from me.

She wore her new shoes out of the store and had worn them just about every day that spring. Seeing my beautiful child with her sparkly shoes made my heart sore. I so desperately missed the life I had before all of this. I bent down and picked Abby up—which made my mom and Kathy cringe, because they were afraid an action like that might make me go into labor. I think I almost gave them a heart attack.

I waddled over to where the chairs were arranged and sat down. Abby followed me and climbed right onto my lap. Kathy tried to take her from me, but she cried and hugged me tightly. My mom tried too and got the same response. She just wanted to stay with her mama. I think that's when everyone realized just how incredibly difficult it had been for me to be away from Abby. To be away from this amazing little person who needed me just as much as I needed her.

After a few moments, my mom stood up and addressed the group.

"I want to thank everyone for being here and helping us honor Crystal today," she said. "We are all incredibly proud of her—the tremendous strength and faith she has shown all along. She's amazing. I don't know how she does it."

My friends slipped a crown of flowers—pink blooms and baby breath—on my head. They also passed out bracelets to me and all the guests. They were decorated with eight crystals—the number of people who were there. That bracelet would come to have enormous sentimental value for me. It would be my "blessed" bracelet—embodying love, faith and hope. I put it on and swore I wouldn't take it off until I had my babies safe in my arms.

I had told myself I wasn't going to cry at this thing. But as soon as the guests started sharing their words of support, I couldn't hold back. Damn hormones.

They said such beautiful things about my strength, faith and hope. They wished me well on the weeks ahead. Everyone was positive about our outcome, predicting that soon we would be home with our baby girls and past this nightmare. I hope you guys are right.

My tears were flowing non-stop. They weren't tears of fear or sadness. They were tears of joy. I was an inspiration? People looked up to me, Crystal Duffy? The love and encouragement my family and friends displayed lifted me up at a time when I so desperately needed it. There were three other women besides myself who were also expecting, not to mention the others who had infants at home. Their words about having strength were a testament to all mothers. As the women continued to offer heartfelt speeches and prayers, there was not a dry eye in the house. My friends and family planned a beautiful celebration to honor me and honor motherhood; I was deeply touched by it.

I returned to my room that afternoon with a feeling that I was surrounded by a loving, calming and spiritual presence. I drifted off into a peaceful slumber.

In my dream, I am surrounded in darkness. I'm sitting in the glider in our bedroom covered with the soft white crochet blanket my mom made me. I have an empty baby bottle in one hand and a pacifier in the other. The babies! Were they finally asleep? I didn't remember putting them back down in their cribs. We were doing a dream feed. I get up frantically to check on them. I'm wearing a thin cotton nightgown, shivering as I close my robe. I walk down the creaky hallway and slowly open the door to the nursery. The room has transformed—it's bigger, and there's a huge bay window looking out the front of our two-story house. Wait a sec, I think, we live in a one-story bungalow. This isn't our house. I'm now standing in my grandmother's old bedroom, her master suite—she has converted it into a nursery for my girls. There's the two white cribs I'd picked out, one on either side of the room. I rush over to them, both Katie and Lauren are in a deep milk-induced coma, each wrapped tightly in a swaddle looking like little burritos. I turn and look around the room, and notice that between the cribs is the changing table that was mine when I was a baby—the one we had used with Abby. It's stocked with their belongings—diapers, wipes, burp cloths and blankets. In the back of the room, there's a daybed. It looks like the Pottery Barn one I always wanted but could never bring myself to purchase. And on it, there she is—my Ita, all curled up, lying right beside Abby, who is clutching her big stuffed doggie. My Ita's short, fluffy, curly brown hair is just like I remembered it. I reach out to touch her and find it warm and soft, reminiscent of newborn skin.

"Ita," I cry out. She opens her eyes.

"Hola mija, vine ayudarte, con las niñas, son tan preciosas."[3]

I couldn't believe my eyes. She is really here, sitting with me in a dream nursery she'd created, telling me she'd come to help with my precious twins. Oh, how I had longed and dreamed for the day I'd get to see her again, to talk to her and have her meet my girls. Ask her all those questions I wish I had years ago when we had the time together. My heart is overflowing with love. For that instant, all the people I love most in the world are in the same room.

---

3   Translation: Hi my daughter, I came to help you with your baby girls, they are so precious.

I'd missed her so much and was so grateful she'd come to meet her great-grandbabies. "*Ay Ita,*" I tell her, "*te he extrañado tanto. Gracias por venir, me hace tan contenta que pudiste venir a conocer a tus bisnietas.*"[4]

As I mentioned the babies, I turn to look back at them, and when I turn back to look at her, she is gone. Our precious moments together were capped. They always were. In this dream and in the many I'd had before. I wasn't sad, but grateful. Grateful that, even if it was for those couple of seconds that I was in deep dream-REM cycle, I got to see her and she got to see me and the girls. I interpreted the dream as a positive sign that we were all going to make it through. That even though Ita wasn't with me in the flesh, she was always around, guiding me, giving me strength when I didn't think I had any left. I was okay. I knew I would be able to carry on. No matter what happened, I felt ready to handle it.

---

4   Translation: Oh Ita, I've missed you so much. Thank you for coming. I'm so happy you were able to come and meet your great-granddaughters.

CHAPTER 19

I'M NEVER GOING BACK

A couple of days later, per Dr. Cooper's request, I was having another bio physical ultrasound so we could get a good image of the girls' positions.

"So, tell me more about your anniversary evening and your baby shower," Ashley said as she smeared gel on my stomach. I was lying on my right side; it had become extremely painful to lie on my back. I faced her in the exam chair and we were catching up.

"It was wonderful. I can't thank y'all enough."

"It was our pleasure. You have really impacted people here, you know. Your positive and cheerful disposition is contagious. If someone saw you on the street, they would never guess all that you've been through," she said as she began her scan on my stomach, her focus alternating between me and screen.

"Thank you. That's so sweet," I beamed.

I felt like the lucky one. To be in this position, extremely stressed and vulnerable, and to have been enveloped in love by everyone I'd met on this journey. It helped me stay strong, positive, focused and calm—which was critical for my babies. As I basked in gratitude, the mood in the room suddenly shifted. I saw Ashley's face grow tense, and she stopped talking. I didn't want to say anything to interrupt her concentration. I shifted around in the exam chair trying to ease my discomfort.

"Can you stop moving, please?" Ashley snapped.

Geez. Was something wrong?

Ashley eyes squinted; she stared at the screen and scribbled notes. She wrinkled her forehead. "Shit," she said, barely audibly.

"Ashley, what's wrong?"

"I don't know. I mean, nothing. Just give me a minute."

As I lay there in the darkened room, terror shot through my body. I bit my lip so hard that I could feel it bleeding a little. Why wasn't she saying anything? I couldn't stand not knowing. I can't stand the silence.

"Please. I'm freaking out," I finally said. "Is there anything you can tell me? Are my babies okay?"

"I'm really not supposed to say, I could get in big trouble. But we have grown close, and I care deeply about you and your babies, like I do all my patients." She paused and took a deep breath, struggling to find the right words. "There's a lot of fluid. I'm not sure why or where it's coming from. I just emailed and flagged this report to Dr. Miller and the team. Let's wait for them to take a look."

Fluid? Did she say fluid? I was having déjà vu. This experience bore a striking resemblance to the ultrasound when the twin to twin disease was first diagnosed. The fluid had been the key indicator that there was something very wrong with the pregnancy and the babies were in danger. Were they in danger again? Had the twin to twin disease come back somehow?

"Can you see the girls? Are they okay?" I wanted to sit straight up so I could have a better view on the ultrasound screen but knew that I needed to try and stay calm and still.

She nodded unconvincingly without looking at me. "No, that's not what's disconcerting. There's so much fluid; it's hard to see them. I can detect a heartbeat but can't tell how they're positioned."

Shit, Shit, Shit! I was breathing heavily but trying not to hyperventilate. I was going to throw up.

Ashley must have heard my breathing change. "It's okay, sweetie," she said. "Let's sit you up. I'll get you a glass of water and I'll call Jenny to help you back to your room."

I could feel that my face had blanched. My body heaved with each breath. I hunched over, hoping that would prevent me from vomiting, at least until Jenny arrived. As Ashley filled her in, Jenny's face contorted in distress. She wheeled me quickly back to my room and helped me lie down on the bed.

"Crystal, try to stay calm, and lay on your left side." Then she literally darted out of my room in search of Dr. Cooper.

I felt it coming. I couldn't stop it. Acidic chunks of food from my stomach had surfaced and were pressuring the back of my throat. Shit! I thought. I'm not going make it to the damn toilet. I hopped off my bed, losing my balance and falling onto the slippery marble floor. My large bottom cushioned my fall.

As I sat there hunched over, I felt my stomach contracting violently. Partially digested pieces of my lunch propelled into the air and splattered all over the floor and onto the lounge chair. I heaved again onto the floor. My throat was sore, and I felt extremely weak. When I knew there was nothing left in me to expel, I pulled myself onto the side of the bed and slowly got up, trying not to slip on my puke. I sat on my bed and reached for the tissue box on the nightstand to clean up the bits that had dribbled onto my lips and chin. My head spun, dizziness had taken hold along with the nausea. I simply couldn't cope with the notion that my babies were in imminent danger and that we could be losing them at this very moment. On top of everything, the damn smell of my own vomit made me woozier.

I dialed Ed at work. He answered on the first ring.

"Crys, what's wrong?"

I was sobbing incomprehensibly. I managed to eke out the words, "problem," "ultrasound" and "fluid."

He knew in an instant the babies were in trouble. And he knew I needed him. "Just relax, lie down," he said. "I'll be right there."

Ed appeared Harry Potter-style in my room. He must have driven like a bat out of hell. "What happened?" He ran to hold me, almost slipping on the vomit.

I tried to explain as best I could, but I was shaking and sobbing uncontrollably.

I rocked back and forth in Ed's arms, taking deep breaths, rubbing my belly and talking to our babies. You girls are okay, right? What's going on in there? Why is there so much fluid? Please give me some kicks so I know you're okay.

The truth was that I hadn't felt any movement in hours, not since before the ultrasound. My last monitoring had been that morning. I had skipped the afternoon session because of the scheduled ultrasound with Ashley.

"It's gonna be okay, Crys," Ed said holding me tightly. "Ashley heard the heartbeats, right?"

I didn't answer. My mind was so overcome with stress it had shut down. Panic had overtaken every part of me; it was in control.

"I'm going to go talk to Jenny. Okay? I'll be right back." Ed ran out the door.

He came back five minutes later. "Jenny left a couple messages for Dr. Cooper. She said she will let us know as soon as he calls back." Ed grabbed some paper towels, wiped up the floor and chair and then pulled the chair next to my bed. He sat there silently rubbing my back as I lie down on my side to ease the pain and nausea.

"Why don't you try and get some rest? I'll stay with you tonight. I'll call your parents, tell them what's going on and Abby can spend the night there."

I shut my eyes tightly, clutched my soft, pink blanket and cried into the creases. Ed turned off all the lights, including the lamp next to my bed. It was dark and quiet, but my heart raced, trying to keep pace with my mind.

In moments of panic, I thought about my Ita. When she was alive, she helped in my deepest moments of despair. I wished she was there. What would she tell me to do? I thought back to the story she'd told me countless times—the story of a traumatic birth. Hers.

When her mother, Micaela, had been around thirty-five weeks pregnant with my Ita, she went to her mother Panchita's house for dinner one evening. She wasn't due to go into labor for at least another three or four weeks and had had a pretty normal and uneventful pregnancy. She was young and had already delivered two healthy babies prior to Ita, so she was unfamiliar with complications that could arise in childbirth. Micaela's mother, Panchita, however, was. She was the midwife in their small town of Linares in Central Mexico. She had served as a doula, a pregnancy and birthing coach and midwife, for over thirty years. Panchita and Micaela were alone in the house. The children were with their other grandparents so Micaela could rest until the baby came, and Micaela's husband had traveled to Mexico City for work. After dinner, Micaela got up to use the restroom and blood gushed from her womb. She started to scream, "*No Dios mio!*" and collapsed onto the floor, clutching her stomach. She was going into pre-term labor. "*Mami!*" she screamed, terrified. "*Ayúdame!*"[5]

Panchita tried to remain calm and stop the bleeding. She filled a bowl with warm water and grabbed some towels from the kitchen and put a blanket and pillow under Micaela so she would be more comfortable. Micaela was losing so much blood that it was hard to see anything. The baby's head crowned; Micaela gave a few hard pushes and Ita emerged. For a few seconds of terror, she was completely blue. Panchita wrapped her up in a blanket to keep her warm, and after a few minutes, she began to cry. Micaela was still bleeding. Panchita needed to focus on her to try and stop it, so she put the baby on Micaela's chest so she could work. But Micaela was fading; she had lost so much blood. She needed a blood transfusion—something Panchita with all her skill and experience couldn't do for her. She tried desperately to save her daughter, but in the end she couldn't be saved. "*Mija!*" Panchita cried out. "*Por favor Dios, No!*" She was on her knees before her daughter, sobbing uncontrollably. "*Por que?*" she cried. Why?

Micaela was so weak, she could hardly breathe a word out. She lie on the floor, clutching her baby, smiling down at her in her arms. With

---

5   Translation: Oh God no! / Mom! / Help me!

her last breath, the last thing she said was "Micaela." A few minutes later, she was gone.

We now know Micaela most likely had a placental abruption; the placenta had peeled away from the inner wall of the uterus before delivery. This kind of event is impossible to know or predict beforehand. It is such a rare occurrence, but one that, if not dealt with immediately, can result in hysterectomy, or worse, maternal mortality. Treatment exceeded the medical capability of rural Mexico in the early 1930s. Micaela had needed a blood transfusion, medical instruments and devices that Panchita just didn't have. Poor Panchita sat there cradling her daughter in one arm and her granddaughter in the other, wailing. She was devastated and heartbroken that she hadn't been able to save her daughter. It was a tremendous feeling of guilt that would weigh heavily on her for the rest of her life. In all her years as a doula, she had never seen anything like the tragedy of her granddaughter's birth. But in the midst of this tragedy, a beautiful, healthy, but very tiny little miracle baby was brought into the world. She grew by the grace of God; every nursing mother in town donated breastmilk for her care, and with her grandmother's love and devotion, she thrived. She was a strong little fighter. Panchita named her Micaela, just like her daughter, and with her husband, raised her like she was her own.

As I lie on the hospital bed thinking about this story, I suddenly felt like I was seeing all the events unfolding before me, but instead of Micaela collapsing on the floor, it was me. But how could that be? What was happening? It was me who had experienced a placental abruption. My body had bled out and no one could save me. Blood stained the floor and my grandma Ita screamed and held me in her arms, begging, pleading and praying for me to come back. The twin babies' cries echoed in the room, but there was no mother to care for them.

I heard Ita's voice. "*Ay, Dios mio, por favor.* Please Lord, please. Don't take my granddaughter. Don't take Crystal from us. We need her here, her babies need her."

I gasped for air. It had been a dream, and now I was awake, coughing. But the dream had felt so real. "No!" I screamed. "Oh God, no."

I startled Ed who had fallen asleep on the freshly cleaned lounge chair. "What's wrong?" he mumbled. Someone must have cleaned more while I was asleep. The room smelled like disinfectant.

Paul came rushing in. "Are you okay, honey? I heard screaming."

I tried to sit up.

"I just had the worst nightmare."

"Oh okay," he said looking relieved. "I was worried that you were going into labor. Dr. Cooper will be here to check on you this morning. Let me know if you need anything," he said, and he left.

I wished Dr. Cooper could have been there right then to comfort Ed and I and give us some reassurance, but we were left alone to deal with the results.

Ed asked again, "Are you sure you're okay?"

"It was just a dream," I told him. I was breathing heavily. "Thank goodness it was just a dream." I rubbed my belly. I still hadn't felt any kicks. Maybe the girls were just sleeping—tired from all the commotion earlier. I hoped and prayed in those minutes that they were still with me.

I'm here, sweet baby girls, I told them. I'm not going anywhere. Please promise me you will pull through again. That you will fight and get through this.

"What happened in the dream?" Ed asked.

"It was about my great-grandmother who died in childbirth when Ita was born. Everything was just as I had pictured it. I had heard the story so many times from Ita. It was in their small town in Mexico around the 1930s, only instead of Micaela dying, it was me leaving newborn Katie and Lauren, and Abby and you."

"Oh, my gosh. Don't even say that." Ed sat next to me and hugged me tightly. "I don't know what I would do if something ever happened to you."

I lie in bed, my thoughts ensnared by this generational pain. Some healers said pain like this could be passed from generation to generation. I knew it was something I was carrying, the pain of my grandmother's birth—and her mother's death—in pregnancy.

He held me until I fell asleep again. Even though I wanted the comfort, I found a small sense of reassurance in the fact that the doctors hadn't rushed in that evening. I knew they had seen the reports Ashley had created and would give us an update first thing in the morning.

When I awoke, it was still dark. I sat up and reached for my phone; it was 6:30 a.m. Ed was curled up on the chair next to me, sound asleep. I grabbed a blanket from the foot of my bed and placed it on him. As I lie back down on my side, I felt little flutters of kicks on my left.

I began to cry with relief. Oh, thank God, I told my girls. Mommy was worried sick! I will hopefully get to see what you two have been up to on the ultrasound screen.

I cried tears of relief, of hope, but also of fear. I was definitely not prepared for the worst, but rather, hoping to hear the best-case scenario from the doctors—that we would be delivering that day.

I heard a faint knock on the door. It was Susan. "Hi," she whispered. "I was just coming to check on you. Paul said you had a rough night and quite a scare yesterday. I'm so sorry." She wrote her name on the whiteboard and then turned back around. "I'm still getting briefed on everything for the day. I'm on duty this weekend for the day shift. Please let me know if you need anything." She grabbed the trash can, which desperately needed to be emptied, and disappeared.

Dammit! I thought. I wanted Jenny to be my nurse. I really needed Jenny. I needed her to help me get through the day. Maybe I could call her to come up. I bet she would.

Susan returned and put the trash can back with a clean liner.

"Do you know when Dr. Cooper will be here? Did he mention a time when he called?" I asked eagerly.

"Usually around 7:00 a.m., maybe a little earlier depending on the rounds. If you're hungry, I'd go ahead and place your order. Sometimes they get backed up on the weekends," she smiled and left my room.

Order breakfast? I didn't think so. I needed to have an empty stomach. We just might be delivering the babies that day. No food or drinks after midnight. That's the standard procedure. I decided I'd just take one last tiny sip of water.

I got out of bed and headed for the bathroom. I turned on the shower and let it run for a minute to get nice and hot. I stepped in slowly. It might be my last shower before the babies were born. I had a strong feeling that that day would be the day.

I anticipated Dr. Cooper saying, "Okay, that's enough. We can't have any more of these scares. Let's do it. Let's deliver these babies and save them while we still can."

Ed, Dr. Cooper and I had discussed the game plan a countless number of times. We all knew that there would come a point where the risks the babies faced in the womb (because of the Mono-Mono status and the cord entanglement) would outweigh the potential risks they might face being born premature. Basically, we'd be taking a lower risk gamble and cashing out, rather than waiting for the bigger gamble and losing everything. There was always a question in this unknown balance. No one knew when that point was. One thing was certain: I wanted to deliver them. I didn't want to keep tempting fate.

After the shower, I blow-dried my hair. Would today really be the day? Will all this pain and fear finally cease? I was so close to thirty weeks. *Please*, I prayed, *let's not risk it anymore.*

I plunked down on my bed. Ed was still asleep. I glanced at my nightstand and saw a note I had written myself earlier that week.

Crystal, be an advocate for your babies.
Don't wait too long. With Mono-Mono twins, you can't risk it.
There will come a time when the risks they face in the womb are
far greater than any potential risks they face being premature.
Remember, the story of the lady in New York.

I knew I really should have stayed off the Mono-Mono twin mom support group blogs. Even with all the wonderful and positive, countless inspiring stories I read, I somehow only remembered the most heart-breaking ones. A few days earlier, I had read a tragic story of twins much like mine. It shook me to the core, and I couldn't get it out of my head. What if this happened to us? We had already come so far. We had to stop gambling with their lives. We needed to deliver them today.

Another tap on my door. Dr. Miller pushed an ultrasound machine into my room. Dr. Cooper and Susan followed behind him. Ed was awakened by the sounds of the approaching entourage.

I knew it, I said to myself. They had all come to weigh in carefully on the obvious course of action: delivery. The more doctors the better; we could just roll on into surgery. And it would be perfect since Ed was in the room too. It was all set.

"Good morning, Crystal," said Dr. Miller.

"Hey kiddo," Dr. Cooper smiled at me. Susan waved sweetly and whispered hello from across the room.

Dr. Miller spoke first. "Our team has looked over the report Ashley sent us. There is an unusually high amount of fluid in the amniotic sac, which makes it more difficult to measure the size of the babies' growing organs." He paused.

Okay, and...?

"We want to go ahead and do another ultrasound," said Dr. Miller sounding concerned.

"I've been freaking out since yesterday. Let's do this," I said. I lifted up my shirt and lie back on the bed.

"That's why we all came, we wanted to see the ultrasound for ourselves," Dr. Cooper said.

Susan slathered cold gel all over my stomach. I closed my eyes and inhaled deeply. Dr. Miller performed the scan while Dr. Cooper, Susan and Ed watched the screen. Dr. Miller glided the instrument all over my abdomen, scanning every square inch.

We heard two heartbeats; their rhythmic pulse was music to my ears. Oh, thank God. But I couldn't make sense of the images on the screen. What in the world are you two doing? I scolded and glanced at Ed who was also trying to discern the images.

"Well," Dr. Miller piped up, "it looks like the girls are wrestling."

"What? That's crazy," I said. "And extremely dangerous. They need to knock it off."

"Those two," Dr. Cooper said shaking his head. "Looks like one baby is lying across the other and their cords are definitely tangled up in there. But everything seems to be fine. Let's just hope this activity doesn't lead to any serious cord compression." He paused and patted my shoulder. "Hang in there," he said.

WHAT? You have got to be flipping kidding me! You are telling me to hang in there when we almost lost them. Our course of action is "let's hope this activity doesn't lead to serious cord compression." Their damned cords are already entangled and they're wrestling in excess amniotic fluid.

"What?" I snapped. "That's it? That's all you're going to say to me, 'hang in there?'" I looked directly at Dr. Cooper. "Aren't we delivering today?"

Dr. Miller replied before he had a chance to speak. "No, there's no immediate threat or reason to."

"But their cords are already entangled and they're wrestling. They're only going to get more entangled, and of course, they will get compressed if we give them the time to do so."

I could feel my face turning bright red.

"For Pete's sake, why are we gambling with time here?"

Dr. Cooper jumped in. "Their cords have been entangled since we first knew they were in the same sac. It was just a question of how entangled, which is why we monitor you."

My head dropped and I placed my face into my hands.

"I have been here monitoring for over a month," I said. My voice was steely. "My entire stay has been endless stress and worries for their safety. I'm almost thirty weeks. Can we please just deliver today? We can't risk their lives anymore."

Dr. Miller and Dr. Cooper exchanged glances. Dr. Miller spoke up first. "No, I would advise against it, Paul."

Dr. Cooper stared back at him. He looked angry. *Was Dr. Cooper on my side?* "Got it, Andy," he said, then turned to look at me. "I'm sorry, kiddo. I know you are disappointed but today is not the day. The babies look fine on the ultrasound. There is no reason to. We will monitor you more often if it makes you feel better."

Oh, man. I could feel my blood boiling. I couldn't hold my feelings in any longer.

"That's it!" I screamed. "I've had it!" I burst into hysterical tears. *Sorry, doctors, but I'm not at all sorry.* "I can't do this anymore!" I sobbed. "It's too much! It's got to stop!!"

Ed pleaded with the doctors. "Won't you please reconsider? We're scared for our girls."

Dr. Miller spoke up. "If you recall what I said in our first consultation, we usually try to wait and deliver ten weeks after the ablation surgery. Or as close to thirty-four weeks as we can get."

"Thirty-four weeks?" I screamed, and then resumed crying.

"No, that's not what we discussed with Dr. Cooper," Ed said.

"Andy, ya'll please, give us a minute," Dr. Cooper said looking at his colleagues.

Dr. Miller, and Susan cleared the room. Dr. Cooper remained with Ed and me.

THIS IS ABSOLUTELY RIDICULOUS, I thought. We had been through so much. We were so close to the finish line. Why couldn't we just deliver? Yes, the babies would be preemies. Yes, they would have to spend time in the NICU. But they'd be alive and there for me to love and support through their struggles. I didn't want another day of stress and anxiety from the unknown. Why did things keep happening, messing with my mind and my emotions? I had long stopped going to the antepartum meetings because our group kept shrinking in size, it seemed as though everyone was leaving but me, spurring envy and sadness.

Had I finally lost it? Why couldn't I just keep it together? My brain, my heart, my soul had been on overdrive for too long. I yearned for my babies to be born so I could end this nightmare. And they wouldn't do it, the doctors just wouldn't do it.

"I'm sorry about all these scares." Dr. Cooper said. "I know how incredibly difficult this is. But trust us, everything looks okay. We are doing well. Let's keep going," he urged me.

I shook my head. "There's no way I'm going to thirty-four weeks. I can tell you that right now."

"I know that's what Dr. Miller is pushing for. Let's just make it to thirty-two and we will talk about it then, okay?" Dr. Cooper said, rubbing my shoulder.

Thirty-two weeks was the magic number. That was when most doctors called delivery for Mono-Mono twins. It was thought to be the time when the risks the babies faced in the womb—cord compression—far outweighed the risks of being premature and spending time in the NICU.

"I've got to get out of here. I need to be outside, to see sunshine and the sky and breathe some fresh air," I sobbed into my trembling hands.

"Ed," Dr. Cooper said, "you can take her across the street. Go grab a bagel or some cookies from Starbucks. Clear your mind. Go take a break."

"No! I don't think you understand. I can't do any of this anymore—the monitorings, being trapped in a hospital bed, the non-stop stressing about whether my babies are still alive. It is way more than one person can bear." I was sobbing and talking at the same time. I didn't know or care if the doctors understood me. I just needed it to be over. I wanted my girls there with me.

Ed grabbed a wheelchair from the hallway and helped me in. He wheeled me down the hallway and down the elevator. When we emerged from the hospital, I felt the sun on my face and the wind in my hair.

I'm never going back, I told myself.

PART 3:

THE DELIVERY

CHAPTER 20

A MOTHER'S INTUITION

The warm summer breeze was blowing on my face. The sun was shining down brightly as we crossed the street. We exited the front doors of the hospital, Ed pushing me in the wheelchair down the uneven sidewalk.

"Eh, sorry about that, Crys." Ed kept apologizing. We stopped outside of the coffee shop—the one that is known as the resident hang out spot. Sure enough there was a line that came out the door all with young doctors, scrub caps on their heads, checking their iPhones. I didn't want to go inside. I wanted to stay outside basking in the warm sunlight and get as far away from the hospital as I could. I had not been outside the hospital walls in over a month. I felt like Morgan Freeman in The Shawshank Redemption where he's just escaped. There was so much I had missed. I hadn't even been fully conscious of it all.

"What can I get ya?" Ed asked as he placed the break down on the wheelchair.

"Açai refresher with lemonade and a cinnamon raisin bagel, toasted with cream cheese," I said as I stared off into the distance.

"Okay, I'll be right back," he said as he pulled out his wallet.

Across the busy intersection on the other side of the hospital, I could see the entrance to the zoo. The parking lot there was beginning to fill up. It was a mild Saturday, not too hot yet for Houston in June. Families were out and ready for fun afternoon adventures at the zoo. To the right of the zoo, there was a small park were all the playground equipment had been beautifully crafted from wood. Engineered wood fiber scattered across the playground. Children were running around playing tag using the big oak tree in the center as base. To the left of the park was a six-mile dirt trail that looped around the zoo—I knew the track well, it went all the way around the University and then looped back around. A young girl, maybe twenty-three or twenty-four, dressed in athletic gear was getting ready for a run. She wore Lululemon pants and an Orangetheory Fitness tank top. She had bright pink shoes, the kind made especially for long-distance runners with extra bouncy soles to support the feet. She wore a navy-blue baseball cap that said Rice Owls and had Sammy their mascot peeking over the letters. No doubt a college student going on a long run before the day of studying ahead. Seeing her across the street brought me back to my own running days. A few years earlier, I had spent months training with a group of friends. We were all committed to run the half marathon, which was held in January every year. We had composed our team in the spring and were committed to stick with it so we could have an impressive time the next fall and be able to qualify for the half marathon. Halfway through our training segments, I had to stop. I was inexplicably getting exhausted and unable to finish even just a few miles of running. I didn't know what was going on. Later that month, I discovered that I was pregnant with our first baby.

I would have given anything to be able to take off running now. Feel the wind in my hair, sweat dripping along the side of my face, an incredible sense of freedom and independence. How long would it be until I could run again? Until I could get those endorphins and natural high from the physical release?

"Here you go, sweetie," Ed said handing me my refresher and a little brown paper bag with my bagel inside.

"Thanks," I told him and took a big sip of my drink. I leaned back in my chair.

"I'm not going back, Ed," I declared.

"What do you mean?" He asked.

"I just can't do this anymore. This is absurd."

He nodded in agreement.

"I know, believe me I know. It's been hell for me, and I can only imagine how incredibly difficult this is for you. But let me tell you something. I've been so amazed with you, so proud of the way you have handled everything. I knew when we met that you were a strong person, but these past few months you've blown me away with your strength and courage." He grabbed my hand and kissed it.

"You are almost there Crys, the girls need you now more than ever... they need you to help them finish their journey," he said.

I sighed heavily. I knew my girls needed me.

When my sister was in high school, she was a bit of a handful, always coming home a few minutes after her curfew and pleading to my parents to stay out longer with her friends. I didn't realize at the time how stressful it is to be a parent of teenagers—the raging hormones causing drastic mood changes. I remember my mom once shared her parenting tip with me.

"I never gave up on your sister. I stayed on her and made sure she did everything she needed to do. A mother never gives up on her children, ever," she said to me.

My mother's words repeated in my head. I said I was never going back to the hospital, and I didn't want to, but I kept thinking about my babies. We were so close. I couldn't give up on them now or ever. A mother never gives up on her children—I thought back on my mother's words.

We sat at the coffee shop for well over an hour, talking, trying to lighten the mood. We reminisced about our past, telling each other funny stories from our college days. I started to feel tired, and I did have another monitoring coming up—that was important for me to do. I asked Ed to take me back to the room.

When we got there, that ultrasound machine was still in the same place. They hadn't removed it from the scan earlier that morning. All the anxious, combative thoughts I had tried to leave outside came rushing back to me. Why wouldn't they deliver my girls?

I kept hearing Dr. Cooper's words in my mind.

"You are doing the best thing for your babies by keeping them in as long as you can." Everyone—Dr. Cooper, Dr. Miller, even Ed, thought that the babies would let us know when they were ready to come, and if they didn't, the doctors would make the decision to deliver them closer to thirty-two weeks.

That was such bullshit.

Later that afternoon, Ashley came by to check on me. The day after our dramatic ultrasound she had become very ill and had to take a few days off.

"Are you feeling better, Ashley?"

"Yes, loads. Everything I catch—whether it's a cold or flu—is a harder recovery for me. But anyway, how are my Duffy girls doing?"

She rubbed my belly and sat down next to me.

"They gave all of us quite the scare."

Just as I was about to go on a rant about my doctors, there was a lively knock on the door; it sounded impatient.

In walked in my doctors—both of them. Oh geez. Glad I wasn't bashing. What could have happened to warrant the presence of both doctors?

"Hi Crystal," they both said at once as if competing.

"What's up, guys?" I said with a grin.

Ashley got up from the chair near my bedside. "I'll come back and check on you later, Crystal."

"Oh, okay." I said.

She exited the room.

"We were making the rounds and wanted to check on you," said Dr. Miller. "How are you feeling? Are you doing a bit better since this weekend?"

I was feeling a bit better, until you showed up, I said to myself. *Now, I'll probably get worked up again.*

"This weekend I had the scare of a lifetime," I said. I was flustered. I could feel my face flushing. "I thought we'd lost one of the babies," I said wiping the corner of my eye.

"Dr. Miller. I've been here for five weeks. It's getting too risky for them." Say it, say it. "I think we need to deliver them now."

"Deliver them?" Dr. Miller looked puzzled. "Crystal, we want you to try and stick it out until closer to thirty-four weeks."

"What? Are you kidding me?" I said. He's out of his freaking mind.

"Andy, we had planned on thirty-two weeks," Dr. Cooper mumbled. It was as if the two had previously had this discussion.

"Thirty-four is our goal, that's what it's always been," Dr. Miller insisted. "The longer we can keep them cooking, the better. Every day, the more they remain in, the lower the risk for other potential problems."

I could feel a surge of tears. This time I didn't bother to hold them back.

I have to advocate for you two. I want you to be mine. I can't bear the thought of losing you, I thought as I rubbed my stomach.

"Look, doctor," still crying, I stared Dr. Miller straight in the eye, "everything I've read about Mono-Mono twins says to deliver around thirty-two weeks. After that, the babies are at a higher risk inside the womb than out. But here's the thing: I don't even know if we should even push it until then. I feel like something is off." I continued, "ever since the ultrasound with Ashley I've felt something was off."

I couldn't quite put my finger on exactly what it was, but a gut feeling deep inside of me had been sounding an alarm.

Dr. Miller didn't flinch at my gaze. "You'll have another biophysical ultrasound with Ashley tomorrow and we will hopefully be able to get a better picture of the babies' size and growth than we did on Friday. I want you to hang in there, my dear." He patted me on the shoulder and walked out before I had the chance to argue further.

I released an audible sigh, and then I turned and made a hard plea to Dr. Cooper.

"I can't play this waiting-for-something-to-happen game anymore. It's terrifying. It seems like everything goes well for a few days—the babies are fine, healthy and kicking away, and then we have a scare that terrifies me to the point where I think I'm on the brink of losing one or both of the girls. We have come so far. They have come so far. I can't help but think that we are being foolish and greedy.

"We are gambling with time, Dr. Cooper," I said. "I still wholeheartedly think we need to deliver soon before it's too late."

Please, I prayed, please, please take my side on this.

He paused for a moment before he answered.

"Crystal," Dr. Cooper said, taking my hand and patting it, "you are doing an awesome job in here, kiddo. This rollercoaster ride of emotions is not easy. We know that, but we just want you to hang in a bit longer. It's almost time." He smiled warmly.

I tried another angle. "I read something online that really freaked me out," I confessed.

"What was it?" he asked.

"I read this story on Facebook," I said. "It happened two years ago in upstate New York. The woman had known early on that she was having Mono-Mono twins—around week nine or ten—because the docs hadn't seen the dividing membrane. They knew they were in for a rough journey ahead. She had a relatively normal pregnancy, as normal as being pregnant with Mono-Mono twins goes. Her doctor had her visit a maternal fetal specialist every two weeks and sent her inpatient at twenty-five weeks—the normal practice. She made it to thirty-two weeks—a monumental victory for a Mono-Mono mom. It was a Sunday; her C-Section delivery was scheduled for the very next morning. During her evening monitoring, everything looked fine.

She fell asleep peacefully thinking the next morning she would safely deliver her babies. Something happened in the middle of the night—the twins' cords became compressed; it must have happened really fast. When she awoke the next morning for her pre-op ultrasound, they couldn't find the babies. She screamed so loud that every patient in the hospital heard. Every nurse and doctor in the hospital came to see her to offer their condolences. All were completely perplexed. No one was ever able to give her any clarity as to how or why it happened. She cried out in anguish and unthinkable pain. Why hadn't her doctors delivered them sooner? Why had they waited so long knowing the risks? Why was getting to the magic numbers of thirty-two weeks and thirty-four weeks so important? Was it more important than the babies' immediate threat—the Mono-Mono status? Everyone was aware of the risks associated with preemie babies and the amount of time they would have to spend in the NICU. But what's worse: preemie or losing your babies?" I paused, picturing that horrifying post, full of images I would never forget: the photograph of the mother kangarooing her tiny dead babies in the NICU and the picture of two tiny coffins side by side covered with white magnolias and roses and a little sign at the bottom. "OUR ANGEL BABIES." ALMOST IN OUR ARMS, ALWAYS IN OUR HEARTS.

I couldn't even begin to imagine that kind of pain, that loss and after having been so close to delivery. Hours before her C-section. Talk about losing my shit…I'd be One Flew Over the Cuckoo's Nest if that happened to us.

"I'm tired of gambling with my babies' lives. I'm done," I told him. "If I could deliver them myself, I would."

"That's a terrible story," Cooper said. "But Crystal, you have to understand we have compelling medical reasons for wanting to keep the babies in. It's not an arbitrary and capricious decision."

"You sound like Ed," I poked a smile.

"I overhead him telling someone that on the phone, I liked it," he smiled warmly.

In a calm and soothing voice, he continued, "Your babies are healthy and doing well in your womb. We don't want to call it quits unless there is an immediate threat. Just try and hang in there a bit longer. We are monitoring you around the clock; we are not going to let anything happen. At the first sign of anything, we will act quickly to get the babies out." He paused and looked back at me. "I can get the babies out in less than two minutes if I need to."

Must be a record time. Still, those weren't the exact words I wanted to hear. My heart sank; my eyes brimmed with tears, making it hard to see. I reached for a tissue. "But Dr. Miller said thirty-four weeks."

"Don't worry about Dr. Miller. You're my patient, and I get to make the final call."

Thanks, Dr. Cooper. I would have liked him to say we were delivering that day, but I did understand his position of looking out for me and the babies and not wanting to act impulsively out of fear.

"I'm going to give you another round of steroid shots for lung maturation—the same kind we did when you were twenty-five and twenty-six weeks," he said.

It was hard to think back that far; so much had happened since then. It was before I had come to the hospital. I was in Dr. Cooper's office— trying not to freak out—as we went over the plan and discussed my long-term hospital stay. Then I had returned to the exam room and the nurse administered my shot, right smack in my booty. It was apparently the most effective spot.

"The statistics are better for us the longer we go. Approximately seventy-five percent of preemies born at thirty-two weeks develop normally without any health problems. There's a 95–98 percent survival rate. And this is just for singletons, not even accounting for twins."

"What about the other fifteen percent?" I feared the answer.

"Well, there are mild to moderate disabilities including blindness, deafness, retardation and cerebral palsy, to name a few."

"Please stop. I don't want to hear any more." I was so over this. Mentally exhausted from thinking (and trying to not think) about all of it. It had consumed me.

I could no longer fight off my worst fears any more. It was as if I had used up all the fight I had left. I knew I wouldn't make it to thirty-two weeks, let alone thirty-four weeks. People speak of mother's intuition—instances where mothers have thought they heard a muffled cry of a child a long distance away or had a gut instinct to check on their kids and were able to save them in the nick of time from catastrophes. This was similar; I couldn't put my finger on it exactly.

I wasn't sure what my little peanuts were up to inside of me, but I had gotten to know them over the last few months. They were strong, active and well, a bit mischievous—poking into membrane holes and tearing them down. But they had been quiet since our last scare. Too quiet. *If only I could convince Dr. Cooper to act before you guys do*, I told them silently. *Please, please don't entangle your cords, baby girls. We are so very close.*

I would try one last time to make my case. "So, will you think about it? Dr. Cooper, would you please consider delivering Katie and Lauren sooner rather than later?"

His pager started to go off.

"Crystal, I'm sorry, can we finish our talk later? I have to scrub into surgery. I'll come and check on you later this evening." He gave me a reassuring pat on the shoulder. "Don't worry; your babies are fine. Hang in there; this will all be over soon." Dr. Cooper adjusted his scrub cap and darted out the door.

I took a deep breath and leaned back on my bed. I touched my belly. *Girls, please stay safe a little bit longer,* I implored, *and throw some extra kicks at your old mama so I know you are okay.*

My mid-morning snack was delivered. Then the cleaning crew descended upon me for their daily rounds of disinfecting the hard surfaces and gathering my laundry. When the morning hustle calmed down, I leaned over and picked up the preemie book a friend had given me. Seventy-five percent chance of survival, ninety-eight percent chance of being born "normal" or without serious health conditions; I just kept reading and going over all the statistics. I took notes on both positions and made two different columns—thirty-two weeks versus thirty-four weeks. I knew that, on paper, we needed to stick to the plan—aim for the goal of thirty-two weeks. Despite Dr. Miller's recommendation, I knew there was no way I could make it to thirty-four weeks.

I dropped the book and surrendered to a deep sleep.

I woke up around dinnertime. It was Ed's night to stay at the hospital. He had brought Mexican food from my favorite place—fajitas, chips and queso and even a virgin margarita for me to indulge. But I couldn't make myself eat a bite. We FaceTimed with Abby, mom and dad in hopes that it would make me feel better. Of course, seeing our sweet little toddler on the video singing and running around, saying, "Miss you, Mama" made my heart turn to Play-Doh. My father's last words were, "Hang in there, *mija*. Those gemelitas will come when they are ready. And don't worry, they are taking care of each other." I smiled as I pictured Katie rubbing Lauren's back or Lauren reaching for Katie's hand to hold.

After our call, Ed got up on my bed and cuddled up next to me. As we watched the latest episode of *Game of Thrones*, I turned over to my side because I suddenly felt sick to my stomach. The pressure—both physical and emotional—was overwhelming, but something else was going on, too. I knew the way I was feeling wasn't quite normal—something was really wrong.

I curled up in pain. "Ed, get the nurse."

"What's wrong? Do you think you are having contractions?" he asked.

"I'm not sure. Something just doesn't feel right."

Ed sprinted to the nurses' station.

Jenny came running in a few seconds later. "What's wrong, honey?"

"I don't know." My voice got scratchy. "I don't feel well. It's like I can't breathe." The words tumbled out of my mouth in a whisper.

Jenny hooked me up to the monitor for the night. She would keep close watch over the reports from her nurses' station.

I closed my eyes. I hoped and prayed that I would find the strength to get through whatever I needed to get through—either this was another scare, or I was in full-fledged labor. I needed to prepare for either.

She tightened the belts over my stomach and tracked the babies. And then she checked the report. "You have a lot of uterine irritability," she said. "I'm going to call Dr. Cooper."

Uterine irritability? Did that mean I was having real contractions? They weren't even that painful. I hadn't labored long with Abby so I wasn't very familiar with the pains of labor, but had heard it described as very intense period cramps. I didn't often complain about aches or pains to the nurses, despite having been locked up for well over a month, so Jenny knew I wasn't exaggerating, and the monitoring machine confirmed our suspicions.

Jenny flew back into the room, holding a bag of IV fluid and her standard-getting-an-IV-started-tools: a tourniquet, gauze, alcohol wipes, medical tape and the wheeled metal stand.

"Dr. Cooper wants me to start you on an IV drip of magnesium to help stop the contractions."

Stop the contractions? Wow! Was this really happening?

"So, she's in labor?" Ed asked.

"Not if we can stop it." Jenny popped a hole in the IV fluid bag and hung it from the elevated wheeled cart on the side of my bed. She sterilized my forearm with the wipe. It felt cool and the smell was pungent and overwhelming. I braced myself for the sting.

"Sorry, sugar," she said.

I took a deep breath. The needle was in, and after a few seconds of stinging, my arm became cool and numb. The sensation flowed down my whole arm. Jenny carefully pulled the needle out, leaving the catheter and tubing in place and taped them securely down. The fluid moved through the tubes and entered my body slowly. My arm looked like something out of a horror movie; it had been picked and prodded for blood draws so many times over the last few weeks. I'd seen lots and lots of needles.

Jenny told me magnesium was called the "drug of the devil" by nurses and former patients who had first-hand experience. After about thirty minutes I could see why. I began sweating profusely; my whole body was on fire. Sweat poured down my face, my underarms and my back. My throat was parched, and I wanted to rip my clothes off just to cool down. I was horribly short of breath. Ed kept chatting, asking me questions and keeping me company. I could barely produce coherent phrases. He brought me water, grape juice—anything he could find. I sucked on ice chips in between large gulps. He stroked my hair—which at this point was a wet, matted mess. He reassured me that it would be over soon. Of course, he probably meant they would stop the IV drip and then we would return to what we were doing before—the waiting game.

On top of everything, I had splitting a headache that felt like someone was drilling a hole in the top of my head. Were they trying to prevent labor by torturing me? Wasn't it enough that I was going to have to 'get over this' when the episode passed and resume the hell that was my norm? Yes, that's exactly what was going to happen. Tomorrow I'd wake up and this would just have been one more scare to add to the list.

It was so disorienting—the magnesium, the sweltering heat, the headache—I almost forgot where I was. I fell asleep with my head tilted to the left, propped on a pillow, and my right arm, with the IV still intact, awkwardly sticking out off to the side of the bed next to the cart. Dr. Cooper must have told the nurses to let me sleep and skip my usually scheduled nighttime monitoring.

The morning light filtered through the tightly closed window blinds. I heard the familiar sounds of nurse shift changes and meal delivery. My mouth felt cracked, my lips chapped and my throat dry. I was soaked in my own sweat-stained sheets, but the room had turned from a sauna to an arctic freeze. I turned to reach for my fuzzy pink blanket, and I felt a tug in my forearm.

"Oh, shoot! I forgot I was still connected to this bloody thing," I said.

"What do you need, babe?" Ed stood up, buttoning his suit jacket. He had already showered and dressed and was gathering his things for work.

"No, I got it. I'm fine. I just want them to take this darned thing off ASAP."

"Yeah, I'm surprised no one has come in to check on you in a while. I'll go ask them on my way out. I love you." He leaned over and kissed my cheek. "Let me know what Dr. Cooper says when he comes in this morning. I'm sorry I have to go, but I have an early client meeting out past Sugarland. I should be able to come back early this evening, around 6:30." I waved goodbye and watched him leave.

When I first arrived at the hospital, I had quickly been able to adjust to so much alone time quite. But in recent weeks, I really started to feel lonely despite having a steady stream of visitors. Close friends and family came daily to visit and drop off treats, and their presence would bring me great distraction. In the past couple of days, though, since the big scare, I'd stopped feeling so resilient. Ed was the one who visited me the most. He had held it together, put up strong familial support while having to keep up a normal front at work, shuffle back and forth between our house and the hospital and then pick up Abby on the weekends and spend quality time with her. I usually didn't cry when Ed left, but now, watching him walk through that door—even though I knew I would see him later that evening—I sniffled and wiped away a few tears. "Don't go," I whispered. But he was already out of sight.

I tried to lean forward to get up and go to the restroom, but I felt a tug in my arm. "Oh damn!" I said out loud. I'd forgotten, once again, that I was still connected to the IV. They could unplug me now; it was over. I wanted to shower and wash off the layer of dried sweat. Perhaps I'd even wash and condition my hair. I picked up the phone and dialed the nurses' station.

"Jenny, I need you," I spoke into the phone.

"Jenny's not here. She just left. This is Shelia, your nurse for the day. I'll be right in."

Jenny had left? She left without saying goodbye? If she had left in the middle of all this, then perhaps that was an indicator that it was nothing to worry about.

The door opened, I expected to see Sheila, but it was Dr. Cooper.

"Hey, Crystal. How are you feeling?" he asked. His tone was very serious. He marched up to the monitor and started examining the reports from the previous night.

"You definitely have a lot of uterine irritability and some contractions," he said, still flipping through the report. "Let's get you hooked up to the monitor right now, so I can see what's going on."

Sheila walked into the room, holding a cup of ice water and some juice boxes. "Good morning," she said cheerfully as she placed them on my over-bed tray table.

"Can you come and get Crystal hooked up?" Dr. Cooper asked her, sounding more authoritative.

She briskly walked over and turned on the monitor. She grabbed the ribbon belts from the nightstand and pulled them tightly around my belly. For once, the babies were easy to find; she got them on the first try. Once again, the babies never seemed to act up when the doctors were around—only the nurses.

Dr. Cooper stared intently at the screen; I didn't see his eyes blink once. I imagined him in his mind weighing all the options. To deliver or not to deliver. I assumed he was going to increase my dosage of magnesium or try something else altogether.

"It's fine, right? It was all just another scare? Are you going to up the dosage of magnesium to see if it helps?" I asked.

"Um, no, actually," he said, "you are having full-blown contractions. The magnesium isn't working the way I'd like it to." His voice trailed off. "I'm not going to administer any more."

"I must've shed five pounds from sweating last night. This junk," I said pointing to the IV in my arm, "is evil." My arm had dried blood from the IV and stung when I moved it. "So, how are we going to stop the contractions?" I asked.

"We aren't," he replied.

I wrinkled my forehead. It seemed I had missed a part of Dr. Cooper's thought process. Our goal had been to stop the contractions, and since the magnesium failed to do that, the only other logical course of action would have been to try another medicine.

"Why not? I'm confused."

"We are having some babies today!" he said definitively.

"What?" My jaw dropped. I was shocked to hear those words come out of his mouth. I was a giant mess—my hair was greasy and matted. I was still half-covered in sweat; my throat was so dry I could hardly talk, and I probably reeked of body odor.

"Are you serious?" I said. "Today? Like right now?"

He turned and looked at me. "Sorry, remind me again, how many weeks are you?"

Dr. Cooper, SERIOUSLY? I thought.

"Thirty weeks and four days." And three hours and thirty-five seconds, but who's counting?

"Okay, yeah, we are definitely doing this."

I was in a daze. I couldn't believe what I was hearing. My mind wasn't able to process the information. All the days, weeks, months of praying and hoping everything would turn out right, that if I could just keep my babies inside me for as long as I could—I could save them. But wait, thirty weeks, that was still so early. It was ten weeks away from full-term babies (not that I ever thought I had a chance of making it to full-term, but still). I remembered those numbers from the preemie book. Just seventy-five percent of babies born at thirty-two weeks developed normally. So what did that mean for us? Was this seemingly wonderful news—the delivery—great news or not? And then I began to blame myself. Maybe if I hadn't said I didn't feel well last night we wouldn't be in this mess. Maybe I'd just be sitting on my bed eating a bagel, watching Good Morning America and waiting for my morning scan. I couldn't believe that this was what I had begged for just yesterday, and now I was questioning myself—my own gut feeling.

I decided to let it all go—the numbers, the statistics, the worries and doubts. I had to keep my faith, hold onto my vision that everything would be okay. And while, yes, I was only thirty weeks along, but...We had been diagnosed with TTTS at twenty-three weeks. I had kept them in for fifty extra days—days we didn't even know they would have when we first learned the severity of the disease. We could have lost them from complications during surgery and any moment thereafter if their cords had compressed. I had successfully made it to thirty weeks. That was a huge accomplishment. Normal or not, who gave a shit? I would love them unconditionally; I was certain of that. I couldn't believe I was finally going to meet them.

I took a deep breath and let it out with a whoosh. *You hear that, girls? Can't wait to meet you on the other side of my womb. Just, don't pull any fast ones during the delivery. Do you hear your mama?*

CHAPTER 21

THE PREP

"Is there someone you want me to call, dear?" Sheila asked. She stood at my bedside and bent down and picked up my phone.

"Shit! Ed! We need to call my husband. He's on his way to the boonies for back-to-back meetings with clients all day." I reached over on the nightstand for my cell phone and pressed the home button, but the phone was dead. Oh no!

"Don't worry," Sheila said. "We will get a hold of him." She was trying to calm me down. "And I can ring your parents too. Their numbers should be in your chart just out here in my station."

"Thank you, and yes," I told her with relief. "Can you get Susan and Paul or Ashley if they are available?"

"Sure, I'll give Susan and Paul a call and tell them to come by your room. Ashley is out sick today."

Sick again? Poor dear.

"Okay great, thank you!"

Shelia advised me against taking a shower since they really didn't want me moving much at that point. I supposed that made sense—I'd probably fall or slip from the nerves. They wanted me calm, relaxed and ready. Only I was far from that. I was filled with stress and anxiety ,and all I really wanted was for Ed and my family to arrive. Sheila brought me a bowl with warm water and a towel so I could wash up. Dr. Cooper had said it would take a couple of hours to get everything ready. Since I wasn't on the schedule they were going to have to do some re-arranging of things. They needed to double-check all the logistics, such as making sure they had an OR to perform the surgery in and to make sure they had enough surgical nurses and staff on hand. My thoughts went back to the countless doctor's appointments that I had during my pregnancy with Abby. After about thirty minutes or longer of waiting for Dr. Cooper in his office, a nurse would usually come in and say something along the lines of, "Mrs. Duffy, I'm sorry, but Dr. Cooper had to run to the hospital for an emergency C-section. One of the other doctors will be in to see you shortly." Well, unfortunately, now I was one of those emergency C-sections. Luckily, there was no need to be stressed or have any reason to think there were any problems. We—I liked thinking I was a big part of that decision-making process—Dr. Cooper and myself had made the call that the morning of June 19 was the time to deliver.

There was a quick knock on the door; it was Susan. "Hi sweetie, how are you doing?"

"Today is the day!" I said with a big smile on my face.

"You are having your C-section? Oh, Crystal congratulations. You must be so excited."

"Yes, I'm still trying to process that this is happening today."

We were interrupted by another knock on the door, in entered Paul.

"What is going on, girl?"

I shook my head and smiled big.

"Today!"

Paul knew what I meant immediately and started jumping up and down.

"Babies are being born today! The Duffy twins are making their debut."

I was laughing so hard I teared up. "Yes, they are."

There was another knock on the door, Sheila and some surgical nurses I hadn't met before came in my room. "Time to get undressed," Sheila said as she held up the sexy backless hospital gown.

"Crystal, best of luck my dear, I'll be praying everything goes smoothly," Susan said as she leaned in and hugged me, then headed out the door.

"Paul, are you available to scrub in?" Sheila asked. "One of our surgical nurses called in sick. There's that hospital flu going around."

"Sure, I'd love to help out with the Duffy twins. I'll go change into my scrubs."

As soon as Paul stepped out it was my turn to get dressed. Sheila and the other nurse helped change me out of my cold, sweaty clothes and into the hospital gown I loved so much. They wrapped a blanket around my shoulders and put socks on my feet so I would stay warm. I still had my wedding ring around my neck on a necklace that Ed had given me. I hadn't taken it off the entire time I'd been there.

"You need to remove all your jewelry," Sheila said. "You can put it in here." She handed me a clear plastic Ziploc bag.

"Even this necklace?" I asked, pointing at my chest. "I always have it on. I'm sure it's okay—it's just a routine C-section."

"Sorry, we still have to follow the protocol, just in case. If something was to go wrong in there, we wouldn't want to have to cut it off or possibly lose it. It's better if we leave it here with the rest of your belongings."

"Okay," I reluctantly agreed and handed the necklace over.

Sheila and the other nurses left. The anesthesiologist, Dr. Williams, came in to ask me some questions.

"Are you allergic to any medications?" he asked in a rough, scratchy voice. He was middle-aged with dark hair, sharp features and a very serious demeanor. Nothing at all like the anesthesiologist I had had with Abby—he'd been a young doctor who had only been at the hospital a little over a year. His wife had just had a baby; he was telling me all about it during the actual procedure. He held my hand

and talked to me the entire time. I wasn't scared. It felt like a long conversation with a friend, with some slight tugging that really felt more like massaging because that area from the waist down was so numb from the anesthesia. "Have you got any names picked out?" he asked and smiled. "We are going to name her Abigail Micaela," I said proudly. When our chat was done, I looked up and saw my big beautiful baby girl. Tears of intense elation came flowing. There wasn't a greater feeling in the world than the high you get from holding your child in your arms for the first time. It's a whirlwind of a moment that comes and goes so quickly, but I was beyond excited to experience it again, and I wasn't going to let this Dr. Williams dude bother me in the slightest.

My parents arrived first. They stayed in the waiting room along with my sister Melissa and Abby. I started to worry. Where was Ed? Was Sheila able to get through to him? I had taken my cell phone off of the charger and had tried to call a couple of times, but his cell was going straight to voicemail. What if he doesn't make it in time? C-sections went so quickly. The doctors have it down to a time. Before you know it, you wake up in the recovery room and it's all over. What if he missed the birth of our babies? I would be devastated; he would be devastated. All the countless hours he had spent with me in that doggone hospital just to miss it.

I started to cry. The surgery prep team barged into my room—no knock—with a "to-go-bed" for me. That was what I called the hospital transportation beds. They were smaller, not as bulky, but way less comfortable than the beds in the patients' rooms. This one had starched white sheets, a blue crocheted blanket and no pillow.

"Can you give me just a minute?" I whimpered.

"Of course," said one of the nurses, the youngest in the group. "We will be right back." They backtracked into the hallway.

Yes, I was a strong girl, but I didn't want to have to do this alone, and I shouldn't have to, dammit. I wanted my husband, my partner, my babies' daddy. My mom and Melissa would have happily stepped in his place, but it definitely wasn't the same. Ed and I were a team. We had been through what seemed like a non-stop string of complications and problems for the past nine months. He should be present for the girls' long-awaited entrance into the world. Why couldn't one damn thing go the way it was supposed to? Why couldn't anything just be easy?

I felt like I had dug up and used all the strength I was allotted in one lifetime. There was none left.

There was a knock on the door. I held my breath, hoping it was Ed. But it was Dr. Cooper, the man-of-the-hour, the superstar, dressed in his bright blue scrubs with his scrub cap tied at the back of his head.

"What's wrong, kiddo?" he asked when he saw the expression on my face and the tears rolling down my cheeks.

"We can't reach Ed," I told him, trying not to sob. "He doesn't know we're having the babies today. His damn cell phone keeps going straight to voicemail."

"I'm so sorry, Crystal," he replied. "Let's give it another twenty minutes or so. I'll let you bring two people in there if you want—anyone you want, your mom, dad, sister. I just saw them in the waiting room. It won't be the same, but you will want someone in there with you."

"Thanks," I said. "When he does get here, I'll be sure to yell at him."

"Okay, kiddo. I'll tell the nurse to keep trying him." And he walked off towards the nurses' station.

The thing was, I couldn't even really be pissed at Ed. He had no idea what was going on. When he'd left that morning, we were both convinced that it had been just another scare, another bump in the road. We thought everything would be the same that afternoon and he would be back in time to have dinner and watch *Mad Men* with me.

Despite the blanket and socks, I was shivering and uncomfortable. My back throbbed and my stomach was in pain too. *Probably just nerves,* I thought.

There was a knock on the door. I was still holding onto that last bit of hope that it was Ed running through the door—in the nick of time. Nope, it was the prep team. *F*ck.*

"Can one of you guys please tell Sheila to grab my mom and sister from the waiting room?" I said. "They're coming into the OR with me."

"I'll go," Paul said as he tied his scrub cap on. There were two other surgical nurses—one right-out-of-nursing-school-young and a seasoned one, a technician and Dr. Williams, the grumpy anesthesiologist. They came towards me like a pack of wolves, and keeping in sync with one another's movements, lifted me up off my bed and placed me slowly down on the to-go bed.

Well, this was it. I was going to have to finish the race alone, without Ed by my side. I'd have to tell him all about it when I saw him again. And then, crazy hormonal paranoia took over my thoughts. Horrific unspeakable things ran through my mind. What if he was dead? *Lying* in a ditch somewhere and not able to get my calls? The stress and anxiety of his absence for the birth had made me a complete hysterical psycho.

"Don't worry, it's normal to be a little nervous before the procedure, but we're here to help you," said the older nurse.

"You don't know shit," I snapped.

The prep team wheeled me down the hall. We turned a corner and stopped in front of the elevators. As Dr. Williams put in his key for the elevator to open, I heard a faint voice coming from far away. *Well, I'm as crazy as Miss Havisham*, I thought, *so it's probably nothing.*

"Oh look," said the older nurse, pointing. Shelia was down at the end of the hallway, waving her arms, trying to get our attention.

"Wait, Crystal, wait!" She was coming to break the news to me that my husband was in fact dead—I was going to be a widow and new mother the same day. I put my head in my hands and started sobbing.

"There's someone else coming this way," said the tech who, until then, hadn't spoken.

I turned and looked back down the hallway and saw a guy wearing a gray pinstriped suit running towards me. It was my guy.

I had never been happier and more relieved in my life. Tears were running down my cheeks. "Ed!" I said. "Oh my God, you are alive! And you are here!"

"Of course! I wouldn't miss it," he said. His cheeks were bright red. He was out of breath and he was sweating so much he looked like he had just run a marathon in the Texas heat. But he had a huge smile on his face.

"Sheila called my office downtown. She got hold of Pat, my secretary, who tracked down the country club I was at with my client. She then called the club and they found the room I was in. Everyone there was so worried about me making it here on time for the birth of the babies."

"I was completely freaking out," I screeched. I almost peed my pants. "I thought I was going to have to do this alone." He leaned in and hugged me.

"I'm here now, sweetie. You won't be alone. I was literally doing 100 mph down Highway 59. Luckily, there was no traffic. I must have had some divine intervention to be able to make it here to you safely and just in time."

Dr. Williams looked down at his watch and then back at us.

"Follow us sir," he said. "You can put on a scrub gown while we administer the spinal tap and the anesthesia. It will actually work out well since some dads have been known to get queasy, even faint, when they see a huge needle being injected into their wife's back."

"Ah excellent." Ed was glowing more than I was. He hadn't known everything I had gone through that morning, but he had gone through an ordeal himself just to be back at the hospital in time. He was going to witness the miracle of childbirth again. Nothing in the world had brought him as much joy as being in the delivery room when our little Abby was first born. Now, he would get to experience that again, perhaps for the last time.

We stepped into the elevator. I had no idea what time it was or if we were running behind schedule. I didn't care. Ed had made it. My sanity had returned and I was calm and ready to have some babies. Let's do this girls!

THE BIRTH

My eyes adjusted to the overly bright fluorescent lights.
The OR room felt more like an arctic resort in Helsinki. There were two
overly bright surgical lights right above me. A stainless-steel table to
my right held sterile tools and instruments. The far back wall was lined
with glass storage cabinets fully stocked with medical supplies. What
caught my eye, and the most important thing in the room, were the two
neonatal incubators sitting side by side. Their sole purpose was to keep
the babies warm and safe when they left my arms to be transported to
the NICU.

It was time for my spinal tap, the magic drug that had come to so
many women's rescue. I looked forward to receiving it. I knew once the
spinal tap and anesthesia were administered, we would have to get the
ball rolling fast—before the medicine wore off.

Dr. Williams approached the foot of my bed, needle in hand, ready
to inject the good stuff. "Lean forward," he demanded. I had been lying
on my back, toes pointed in the air, exposing the brightly-colored footie
socks the nurses had put on me. To my right, one of the OR nurses who
had been on standby until she could assist stepped up. Young, with a
soft face, golden blonde hair and freckles on her cheeks, she grabbed
me by the side and helped me sit up all the way on the bed. It took an
extraordinary amount of effort. *Why didn't they just use the same type
of bed like the one in my room?* I wondered. Who knew? The hospital
had standard procedures and idiosyncrasies. This was probably the
latter. I hunched forward on the bed with my gown pulled open in the
back and tried not to think about what my squashed butt looked like
under the bright fluorescent lights of the OR. Without so much as a
warning, Dr. Williams jammed the needle between the spinal bones in

my lower back. At first, it felt I was being stabbed and then nothing but pain. I twitched at the uncomfortable feeling.

"You need to hold still or it won't take," he snapped. Dude, I'm trying, I told him silently.

"Here let me help," Paul said as he took my arms and pulled them forward until my body was curled in the shape of a "C." It felt like a painful yoga pose. Paul hugged me to help keep me from moving. Williams stabbed me again, and this time it worked.

When I got the spinal tap with Abby, I was scared because I didn't know what to expect, and I jumped up off the bed. The movement caused my young anesthesiologist resident to mess up. One of the surgical nurses walked over and gave me a huge bear hug and kept me still so that he could try again. I guess I was still a jumpy gal.

Once the drugs were administered, Paul helped lay me down carefully on my back. The anesthesia machine was at the head of the operating table with tubes connecting back to me; that was where Dr. Williams was hanging out. Paul inserted a catheter, which I couldn't actually feel, but I saw the clear plastic bag dangling over the side of the bed. Goldie put up the curtain—a blue fabric screen—right above my neck, obstructing my otherwise front row seat to my own birth show. Then, Goldie moved to the other side of the theatre curtain and raised my gown all the way up, exposing my naked body which was sprawled spread-eagle. No matter how many babies you had, a room full of strangers looking at your seven-months pregnant body extended on the surgical table was still awkward. Ah, screw it, I decided. We'd overcome a lot of crap to be there. My girls were about to be born, and this pregnancy would soon be over.

The drugs had definitely kicked in. There was a wave of warmth running through my lower body. My legs tingled like pins and needles were going through me, and then, just like that, they went dead. I was loopy and dazed, then became nauseous. I could no longer see Dr. Williams, but he was right behind my head.

"I'm gonna puke, people!" I screamed, getting everyone's attention.

"Here's a bucket," Goldie said as she grabbed a plastic tub and held it up to my face.

My stomach contracted violently and I leaned forward and propelled vomit. Some made it into the tub, the rest splattered on the floor.

"Sorry. That came up really fast." I apologized. Some had gotten on Goldie's sleeve.

"Don't worry," she replied. "It's completely normal to feel nauseous from the anesthesia."

"Let me get you something that might help," Dr. Williams said. He handed Goldie a tiny plastic cup with a little white pill inside.

"Here," she said and popped it in my mouth. "This Zofran should do the trick."

I heard Ed's voice. "Crys, are you okay?" He finally emerged from the back wearing a blue scrub shirt and pants.

"Fine, just a little nausea. It's not my first rodeo." I winked.

"True, but it may be the last." Ed said.

"We'll see. When are you taking me back to Paris?" I joked. It was definitely the drugs talking. I had so much anesthesia pumped in me that I actually thought it would be a good idea to try having more children after this.

"Are we ready to have some babies or what?" Dr. Cooper strutted in confidently. The side conversations of the nurses and tech ceased quickly. The room got quiet as the rock star took the stage.

"Yes, we are!" Ed hollered, raising up our arms together.

He walked up and gave Ed a warm handshake. He bent down close to my face and put his hand on my surgical shower cap.

"Just lie back and relax, and in a few minutes, we get to meet the Duffy twins."

"Relax," I said. "I think I've become an expert in that."

Dr. Cooper was standing over the table with all the medical instruments, surveying them to make sure he had everything he might need. He looked up at Ed and me.

"Oh, and this is pretty cool, I talked hospital PR and they want to do a piece on you and the girls when this is all over."

"Aww, that's so nice," I said. "If I make it through this alive, I would love to share our story with the world."

Everything was coming together exactly the way I knew—or rather hoped—it would. Maybe things were finally falling into place the way they were meant to.

Ed squeezed my hand and bent down close.

"I love you—all my girls," he whispered.

We waited patiently for the surgery to begin. Five of Dr. Cooper's partners—other attendings—had scrubbed into surgery. They wanted to see—hopefully be asked to help—in this delivery of Mono-Mono twins. Only one other doctor had been present when Abby was born—it was been a pretty routine C-section. This time, between Dr. Cooper's staff, some of Dr. Miller's staff, the OR surgical team and each of the girls' NICU teams, there was a massive entourage that crowded the room. I wondered if we would get to see just how tangled the girls' umbilical cords had gotten—how entangled they had been.

The overhead surgical lights blinded me, and all I could really see was the blue curtain separating Ed and I from everyone else on the other side. There were conversations going on between Dr. Cooper, the other doctors and the nurses—but it all sounded like buzz, and I couldn't make out any specific words. I was thankful for that.

The procedure began quickly. There was no formal announcement of the first uterine incision, but I knew it had been made—there was lots of movement behind the curtain. Ed, who was still holding my hand at my bedside, kneeled down. My palm was sweaty, but the nausea had more or less settled itself. I felt like I reeked, though, and I had a terrible itch on my nose. The darn histamine reaction from the drugs. It was relentless, and there was no way I could scratch it. Right as I was about to ask Ed to help me out, I began to feel a tingling sensation in my stomach and pelvic area. I felt breathless, like someone was pushing on my chest—the spinal tap was working. I started taking deep breaths, still holding onto Ed's hand. The image of Dr. Cooper and another associate, Dr. Jones, on either side of my bed pulling and tugging will forever be ingrained in my head. It was like someone was rummaging around in my purse, only the purse was my stomach. No pain, just the odd sensation of a numbed massage.

"Quite a lot of blood here," I heard Dr. Cooper murmur. "Can we get some suction to get a clearer look?" That sounded unnerving, but fortunately, Dr. Cooper immediately added, "the babies are fine, don't worry."

In a voice not much louder than a whisper, I heard him tell Dr. Jones, "Good call to deliver today. This is crazy, huh." I felt loopy. Ed had let go of my hand momentarily to snap some pictures with his cell phone.

"Psst, Ed, what's going on?" I asked.

"I'm not quite sure." He paused to put his phone down and took a few tiny steps forward.

He was shocked at what he saw. "There's a lot of blood, and they are trying to take care of it."

A lot of blood? Hmm. I didn't think that sounded normal. I thought at this point that Dr. Cooper would've been flinging babies at us and putting my uterus back in place.

I looked back up and saw the continued effort of Dr. Cooper and Dr. Jones pulling—quite literally—my stomach apart. *Okay, this must be it,* I thought. Here we go, girls. I was ecstatic. We were seconds away from meeting our babies.

They continued to pull, stretching the walls of my uterus, making space for the babies to come out. It was the weirdest sensation ever. Ed had talked about how they had done this when delivering Abby. He said it was this ripping apart of my abdominal muscles with brute force—not cutting with precise instruments—that had been the most shocking visual image of the delivery for him.

I couldn't see shit, but Ed was giving me a play by play. The bed started to shake. It was very strange. They were high up in there manhandling me, and I didn't feel a damn thing. The bed was shaking so much it was almost funny. Geez, if they pulled any harder they would break the bed. Still no pain, just the slight pressure and touching. Bizarre.

I heard crying. I gave a long exhale at the sound of the long-awaited cry. Sometimes C-section babies don't cry because there is a lot of junk in their airways due to the fact that they weren't pushed through the birth canal. Luckily, that was not the case with us. Whoever came out first was screaming bloody murder.

It was Katherine who was first. Dr. Cooper held her up as if she was the Heisman Trophy and said, "Here's baby A." I let out a huge cry of relief. She was tiny—really tiny—like a child's doll. I had mentally prepared for that, but it was still shocking as hell to see a baby as small as a cabbage. I kept imagining a big, nine-pound, fully-developed baby like Abby had been. She was Smurf blue, but fortunately, she'd come out crying (or screaming, rather). Proof that there was nothing wrong with her lungs—that was for sure.

"The operating room is too cold for her. Put her into the incubator," said one of the NICU nurses. They passed her off right in front of me without so much as letting me hold her or give her a kiss. *What the hell?* I thought. *Bring me my baby, bitches.* But, I couldn't speak.

Less than twenty seconds later, Dr. Cooper held up Lauren and said, "And here's Baby B, folks." Oh, thank God she was out safely!

The NICU nurse grabbed Lauren. I got a "drive-by view" of her, but then the NICU teams blocked my view completely. I was about to lose it. They f*cking did it again.

"Katie! Lauren!" I screamed. My voice was cracking—quieter than I wanted it to be—as I called out for my babies. "Can you bring them to me?" I croaked. But nobody paid any attention. Could they not hear me? Almost robotically, a nurse began to place Lauren in her little bed in the incubator right beside Katie.

"Excuse me," Ed interjected. "Can we see our babies?"

"I'm sorry, folks, we have to keep them in their incubators where it's warm while we check their vitals."

"Yes, but I just want to see them," I said. "Really quick and then you can take them if you must. Please bring me my babies," I pleaded.

"Come on. Can't you bring them over so we can see them?" Ed asked again.

The nurse shook her heard. "We need to tend to their needs immediately. We don't want to stress them any more than we already have with the birth," she said.

"But I'm her mom, and I just want to see them!" I sobbed.

"I understand, and you can see them up in the NICU, ma'am." She took the break off of Katie's and wheeled it out the door. She turned back and said to me, "Oh, by the way, congratulations on the birth of your daughters."

I was devastated. I know there were rules and procedures that the NICU nurses had to follow. Things they had to do to ensure the safety of the babies as soon as they were turned over into their care. But I was their mother. I'd just given birth. This damn nurse was so fixated on checking off the items on her duty list that she failed to show any compassion or human decency and let me meet my babies. Katie was gone. I'd been dying to meet her for months, and she was gone.

The nurse that grabbed Lauren from Dr. Cooper was still standing there. Her jaw had dropped as she'd witnessed the baby snatching-event. She smiled at me. She must have felt compassion. Either that or she was a mother herself and knew—knew that the moment when you see your baby (or babies, in my case) for the first time is the part that makes everything else not just okay, but perfect. And so, she bent the rules and came to me slowly, carrying Lauren in her arms, wrapped in a little blanket.

"Meet Baby B. I'm so sorry, I'm not sure what their names are."

The nurse held Lauren up to my face. She was tiny, wrinkly and pink, and all wrapped up in her little blanket.

"Oh, my goodness," I whispered. "Hello little Lauren. I'm your mama. I've been waiting to meet you for so long."

Lauren started to squirm, she looked right at me and I smiled at her.

"Can I hold her, just for a minute?" I asked the nurse. I knew I was probably pushing my luck.

"I'm so sorry, Mrs. Duffy," the nurse said. "We really need to take her into her incubator. Her temperature is dropping. Little preemies like her usually can't breathe on their own and need to be put on the ventilator for help. Plus, we don't want to stress her much longer than we have to."

"I understand," I said, choking out the words, then mouthed, "Thank you."

She smiled back at me and nodded.

"Congratulations, Mr. and Mrs. Duffy," she said as she placed Lauren back in the incubator. She slowly pushed her incubator in the direction of the door.

Watching her go gutted me. I didn't think it was possible for a person to feel so much pain in their heart. I saw seeing my babies for the first time here in that room, on the other side of my womb, and then a moment later they were gone. That moment of holding them in my arms that I'd dreamed about countless times had been taken away from me. And it all happened so fast, before my mind could even keep up with it all.

I cried. I cried because I was heartbroken. I cried because I wasn't the one right there by the babies' side as they were being poked and prodded by the NICU nurses. And I cried because I mourned the loss of those special first minutes together.

Ed was silent. He was right there by my side, hugging the left part of my arm. I saw a tear trickle down his cheek as we shared a moment of mutual heartbreak. And then we heard Dr. Cooper say, "She's still bleeding y'all. We need to get this under control." His voice sounded mad.

Dr. Williams re-appeared and put his hand on Ed's arm.

"Sir, I'm going to need you to clear this area," he said.

"What in the world?" Ed said.

Dr. Cooper peeped his head over the curtain.

"Crystal has a lot of internal bleeding, we may need to do a blood transfusion," Dr. Cooper said.

The room was silent.

"Back up, clear this space," yelled Dr. Williams.

"Ed, I'm sorry, but we need you to step outside," Dr. Cook said.

CHAPTER 23

PLACENTAL ABRUPTION

It was bright when I awoke; my vision felt hazy as my eyes adjusted to the room. *Am I dead?* I thought. *Where Am I?* I was lying flat on a bed with crisp, white sheets folded up to my neck. The room was dead quiet I was surrounded by three blank walls and a closed curtain. I felt groggy, disoriented and nauseous. I started scanning the room trying to locate a trash can because I felt another puke session coming.

"Hello?" I called. "Ed? Mom? Dad?" I could hear muffled voices behind the curtain.

"Hello? Where the hell is everyone?"

I heard footsteps walking towards me. An older nurse with shoulder-length brown hair pulled the curtain open.

"How ya feeling?" she asked in a soft and gentle voice.

"Like I've been hit by a bus," I told her. I pulled my hand up to my face to massage my temples and felt a tug.

"Ouch, this darn IV." I looked down at my hand. There was dried blood all over the back of my hand and tape strips going every which way to hold the IV in place.

"Where is everybody? My husband, my mom, my daughter?"

"They are in the waiting area, I sent them there so you could rest. Besides, little visitors aren't allowed in the recovery area."

"She's not a visitor," I rolled my eyes, "she's my daughter!"

I wanted to see Abby and Ed. Their presence would calm me and help me get reoriented from my post-surgical, drug-induced sleep.

"I just want my family. Can you please get them?"

"Of course, you will want them near as you've had quite the traumatic day. I'm glad you are okay," the nurse said, she looked relieved.

"What are you talking about?" I wrinkled my forehead and looked at her in confusion.

"You mean, you don't know what happened?" she asked confused.

"All I remember is my babies being born and taken away from me. And then the mean anesthesiologist guy kicked Ed out of the room. Wait, why did he ask Ed to leave? Are the babies okay?"

"Dear, I'm going to let your doctor know that you are awake and wanting to speak with him regarding your procedure. I'll get your family too." She made a beeline for the door before I could get another word in.

"Wait," I cried out knowing no one could hear me. What the hell happened in the OR?

I laid in bed trying to run through basic facts. "Okay, I'm twenty-nine years old and the year is 2014. Barack Obama is the President in office."

I scanned the room again for a trash can. I saw one, but it was at the foot of my bed.

Oh shoot, there was no way I could reach it.

I'm hoping breathing heavily helps my nausea subside. I woke up that morning expecting everything to have all been another scare, just another frightening bump in this rollercoaster of a pregnancy. And then my C-section was scheduled for that morning, and I didn't know if Ed would even make the birth of his own twins. My babies had been born. They were screaming (quite powerfully might I add) and crying. I had heard them, hadn't I? Were they okay? Did they get warmed and plugged into the incubators? With every fiber of my being, I hated the post-delivery procedure for preemie babies: the nurses scoop them up and take them away without so much as a stop to allow their mother to hold, see or kiss them. I wanted to see my babies. Katherine and Lauren—these two little girls had held on strong and fought hard for their lives on multiple occasions throughout the past seven months. These girls tore down membranes just so they could be near each other. These girls had already made a huge impact on my life. Being their mother would be the greatest blessing and honor of all.

I had finally given birth to these little girls that I had dreamed about meeting for months. And yet, I met them so briefly, almost in passing. I have had meaningless conversations with complete strangers on the street that lasted longer. I wanted to see them again. I wanted to hold them close to me, breathe them in and have them lie on my bare chest. I wanted to have them hear my heart beating from the outside. I knew they were going to need my love and encouragement to get through their journey in the NICU and whatever else lay ahead.

I remembered those brief seconds where I had seen them in the flesh. They were tiny and delicate, in need of immediate medical attention. There had been—in those minutes before chaos descended—a strong push from the NICU nurses to get the girls in their incubators and into the NICU. I felt a chill run up my spine as I wondered whether the girls were okay.

The door opened and I heard the sound of footsteps. Then, the curtain opened and revealed my family—a whole big group of them. Ed was there, along with my mom, Melissa and Aunt Eva who held two little plush, pink teddy bears and a shawl. She draped the shawl over my shoulders and hugged me tightly.

"Crystal!" My mom shrieked, ran to my bedside and started hugging me.

Melissa stayed at the foot of the bed, hugging my legs, waiting her turn to tackle me with love.

"*Mija*, we were so worried about you," Eva said.

"We are just so glad you are okay," Mom sobbed hysterically into my shoulder, and Ed came over and kissed my hand.

I looked up at him. "What's wrong?" I said. "What's going on?" I needed some answers.

"We will give you guys a few minutes to talk," Melissa said as she grabbed my mom and aunt and headed out the door.

"I'll be back, *mija*. I just had to come see you—make sure you were really here," my mom said, sniffing into a tissue. Her eyes were filled with tears. And then Ed and I were alone.

"Where's Abby?" I asked.

"She's with your dad in the waiting room. The nurse was being all anal-retentive and wouldn't let us bring her back here."

"Damn hospital policies," I said. "If I ever make it out of here, maybe I'll advocate for that one day," I said.

"Ha, you should. You'll hopefully be able to see Abby when you are settled back in your room."

"Ed," I said, "what the hell is going on? What happened? Everyone is acting a little weird."

"Crys," he said, and then he choked up. He bent down and flung his arms around my neck, holding onto me tight. Then he kissed my cheeks and pecked at my forehead, stroking my hair (which probably reeked of vomit). He couldn't seem to find the words.

"Ed, I'm okay, I'm right here," I said, trying to comfort him.

"Crystal, you almost died," he cried. And for the third time in the decade-plus we'd been together, he cried.

"What?" I said, shocked.

"We almost lost you."

"What?" My eyes widened in fear.

"You had a placental abruption, which basically means the placenta separated from the uterine wall. They didn't realize it was happening until they had started the procedure. When they made the first incision to get to the babies, they saw a lot of blood. There was tons of it, and they had to act very quickly. They got all hands-on-deck—Dr. Cooper, Dr. Jones, Dr. Bernstein and even a couple of their residents. And probably ten nurses. Even before the babies were out, they knew that something was wrong."

I tried to recall the details of the birth exactly as it had occurred a few hours before, but I was blanking, except for one clue something had gone wrong.

"And then Dr. Williams, the anesthesiologist, he made you leave," I said.

"You lost so much blood, they were trying to prepare for a blood transfusion. Clear the way meant they wanted clear access to you in case they needed to call the blood transfusion team. They wanted me out of the way so I wouldn't freak out in there, and also because they needed all the space around you for the dozen doctors who were getting ready to further operate on you."

"I can't believe what you are saying," I told him. I was nearly speechless with shock.

"The waiting itself almost killed me," Ed said, his voice thick. "After they kicked me out of the OR, I was terrified. I didn't know what the hell was happening with you or the girls. I was in the hallway. I didn't want to be in the waiting room with all our family freaking out. I needed to be alone. About twenty minutes after I got kicked out of the OR, Dr. Cooper finally came out," Ed said. "He took his scrub cap off and put his hand on my shoulder. I feared the words that would come out of his mouth.

He said, "Ed, Crystal has suffered a placental abruption. She lost a lot of blood. We had to act very quickly, but she's stable now."

The words pierced my heart.

"I had been so deathly afraid of losing you, I had never prayed so hard for anything in my life. I ran to the waiting room and explained to your family what had happened. They had no clue any of that was happening. I just wanted to see you and make sure you were okay, but the nurse told us to wait and let you rest—she would come get us when you woke up," Ed said.

My mind once again ground to a standstill. I'd reached my capacity for terror and fear and felt like I was temporarily out-of-order. I couldn't even think of questions to ask.

"So I went looking for the babies. They had taken them to a room on the same floor we were on. I went towards them, cell phone in hand, I was ready to get some great pictures and videos, documenting their first few moments of life for you to see. Katie peed all over one of the nurses; she laughed. "Looks like the plumbing works," she said. It was a bit of a comic relief following the scare I had with you. I snapped a ton more pictures of the nurses holding the babies, measuring and weighing them. Then the mood in the room quickly changed. Lauren started projectile vomiting blood. The nurses were scurrying around and whispering. I heard them saying, What's her heart rate? *Call* upstairs and tell them we'll need *thirty* ccs of something."

I felt weak and light-headed with all of this information being thrown at me. I rolled over to lie on my side.

"Immediately, they placed Lauren back in the incubator and pushed her out. They were making a dash up to the NICU.

"'Sir, we need you to step away and out of the room, please,' they told me. They were like military forces mobilizing for battle. In a few seconds they were down the hall and inside the elevator."

Ed paused for a moment.

"And then what did you do?" I screeched. I was crazed with the suspense. I needed to know the end to my own life story.

I looked into Ed's bright blue eyes as he retold the fear he had lived just hours before. They were wide and teary.

"I tried following the girls up to the NICU. Hoping that, if they didn't let me in the room, there might be a window I could peek into, like the nursery when Abby was born. This was not the case up in the NICU. The nurses stopped me at the check-in desk."

"What do you mean they stopped you?" I interrupted.

"I told them I was the Duffy twins' father, and the nurse said I couldn't come in. The babies had suffered some trauma and they were trying to stabilize them. They directed me to the waiting area and said they would come get me with updates."

"Oh my gosh!" I shrieked. "Well, what happened to them? It was because of the abruption, I'm sure." I was freaking out. All this information was too much for me to take. I felt like I was going to throw up at any second.

"So, after being kicked out of the OR with you and then again with the girls, I was freaking out," Ed continued. "It was hell, the worst twenty minutes of my life. I went back downstairs to the waiting area near the OR. The minutes dragged on. So many things ran through my mind. What if you had died? What if our babies died? Would I have to raise our daughters alone? I don't know what I would do if something happened to you. But then Dr. Cooper came out—saving me from a complete panic attack—and told me that they stabilized you, but you were still unconscious. Then, he told me what happened. Usually, when placental abruptions occur, they are more obvious. There is a gush of blood alerting the doctors that they need to operate immediately and get the baby out ASAP. But, in your case, there was no external bleeding—everything was internal, and that made it much more dangerous. If they had tried to give you more magnesium and held off trying to get the babies out, there's a good chance that you and the babies would have died."

It was difficult to wrap my mind around my potential death. Maternal mortality in 2014? It was unbelievable. The undetectable, untraceable placental abruption. I closed my eyes and thought back to that morning. I hadn't eaten anything since dinner and my breakfast was untouched. "I don't feel good." I had told Jenny, my nurse. I remembered pointing to the spot above my abdomen—just above my sternum—close to where I felt the stabbing sensation. I knew something had been happening inside my body. I knew I needed to insist on delivering the babies. It was my body, and I was the only one who knew that something was wrong. All the while, the hospital team—my doctors, nurses, caregivers—had gone to great measure to adequately prepare for our preemie newborn babies, anticipating that they would go to the NICU, but they had been unprepared for a maternal emergency with me. What if I hadn't spoken up? What if I had just ignored my gut feeling in favor of my doctor's years of experience? What if my complaints had fallen on deaf ears who thought the pain I was describing was normal of twin pregnancy and disregarded me? We would have had a very different outcome.

PART 4:

THE NICU

THE UPDATES

Ed and I sat on my bed holding each other tightly, trying to process what had just happened. We heard the door open. Footsteps approached. The curtain opened and there was Dr. Cooper.

"Hey kiddo, you doing all right? That was intense," he said. He took off his scrub hat and took a seat on the bed right beside us.

"I have so many questions for you," I said, my voice choking.

It was hard to find the right words.

"Why?" I said and began sobbing. "Why did this happen to me?" I buried my face in my hands, wiping away tears.

"I'm sorry kiddo, I wish I had an answer for you. The truth is, we don't know. What I can tell you is that your placenta deteriorated. It shredded and completely detached from the uterine wall. We were all shocked as hell. Especially since it was undetected and you hadn't experienced any bleeding," he explained.

"But I was in the freaking hospital!" I interrupted. "I just don't understand. How could this go undetected while being hooked up to all the monitors and everything?"

"The monitors could only detect something if the abruption had already impacted the babies—which it hadn't yet," he said. "Your gut feeling and your persistent contractions meant it was time to deliver. About twenty percent of the time when this occurs, the hemorrhage is concealed, so the diagnosis is delayed, and in some very unlucky cases, unknown until it is too late. In these cases, the fetus is almost always dead. Thank God this wasn't the case for you. I'm so glad you spoke up, Crystal. Heck, I'm glad for all the times you argued or questioned me. All that mattered was making sure you and the babies were okay."

My head was spinning. I kept taking deep breaths in and out—as if physically trying to take it all in. I was trying hard to not start bawling uncontrollably again. I wanted to hear all of it, I needed to hear all of it. I was a mess—emotionally, hormonally, physically, mentally—yet I still wanted to know every detail. How weird was I? It was because I knew I needed to understand everything fully in order to be able to move past it. In depth knowledge equated to healing.

"Crystal," Dr. Cooper added, "this is also extremely rare. It happens in one percent of all pregnancies and chances are even lower with twins."

"So," I said, "it's rare even among twins, yet we still managed to have that happen too."

Dr. Cooper cleared his throat and then put his arm around me and tried to comfort me, but I was beyond comforting.

"And there's no reason for it? What are the causes?" I asked.

"In the past, placental abruption was thought most common in older women, or women of lower socioeconomic status who had been malnourished or had multiple pregnancies, like five or more. Others think a common cause of abruption is drug and alcohol use. This didn't make much sense because none of those things apply to you," he said.

"Also…" he looked away from me, then continued in a very serious voice. "placental abruptions are one of the primary causes of maternal mortality, and those that survive…" his voice trailed off, "sometimes need a hysterectomy because of the severe internal damage."

He paused for a moment, then smiled sweetly.

"You are so incredibly lucky, kiddo. You lost a lot of blood, but we were able to manage it quickly and effectively."

And then he added, "Everything still works in that department, should you and Ed want more children."

This was an absolutely terrifying thought. "Nope I'm good with my kiddos, I need to focus on the ones still here. When do I get to see Katie and Lauren?" I asked frantically.

"Crystal," Dr. Cooper said. I could tell by the tone of his voice that I wasn't going to like what he was about to tell me. He stood up and put his hand on my shoulder. "I want you to rest. You have been through major surgery and a very traumatic birth."

"Rest?" I yelled in annoyance. "But I want to see my babies!" I started to cry.

"Can you take me to see my babies, please?" I pleaded.

"Can we get a wheelchair so I can take Crystal up to the NICU, just for a second, so she can see the girls?" Ed asked.

"I'm so sorry Crystal," Dr. Cooper said, looking down as he pulled out his cell phone.

He scanned through his messages and then raised his head.

"The babies are in the best care right now, and it's my job to care for you. You are still hooked up to the catheter—there's no way you can move today. I want you to rest here for a couple of hours, or until they have your room ready for you."

"My room ready?" I snapped. "Can't I just go back to the room I've been living in for five weeks?"

"Oh, right, yes," Dr. Cooper said. "I want to make sure you are okay and there are no major issues resulting from surgery. Then the nurse will take you back to your room, and in the morning, if you are feeling up to it, you can get a wheelchair to ride up to the NICU." He turned to look at Ed.

"Take care of her tonight," he said, "and please let me know if anything comes up."

He leaned in and rubbed my shoulder, then walked out. I grabbed my pillow from behind my head and flung it across the room as hard as I could. It landed on the floor next to the trash can.

"I just want to see them," I whispered into Ed's arms.

"I know, me too." Ed said.

I couldn't believe I had to wait even longer to see my girls, the precious little twins I'd loved from the moment they were conceived. We had been together every step of the way on this high-risk pregnancy. I realized, in the last week leading up to their birth, that they were the babies I had lost in my two miscarriages. They were the two babies I was always meant to have. They were here not because of one miracle, but because of a string of miracles. By the grace of God and a team of highly skilled doctors and nurses—we were alive. All three of us. Envisioning holding my babies helped me drift into deep sleep.

A couple of hours later, when I opened my eyes, I instantly knew where I was—back in my old space of familiarity and comfort within the hospital. The blinds were half open. It was dark outside, yet you could still hear the cars honking and traffic in the streets. The lamp was on and the curtain had been drawn closed; my plush, pink blanket was draped over me. How strange it felt to be back there and not pregnant. What did I expect? To give birth and immediately pack my bags and run out the front doors? To place the twins in their car seats and head home? I hadn't really given much thought as to how alone I would feel without them inside me. Yes, there were the doctors, nurses, techs, Ed of course and the constant stream of visitors, but my babies we not there. They had been a part of me for so long. The pain of being without them was unbearable. I thought non-stop about my babies: if they were okay, if they were breathing on their own. I thought about how much I just wanted to hold them. I'd been counting down the minutes until the morning—when I hoped they would remove the paralyzing catheter— so I could get up and walk over to the NICU to see them.

I felt myself approaching the state of *One Flew Over the Cuckoo's Nest*. I was well aware that mothers are usually a bit emotional and hormonal; they get a case of the "baby blues" after giving birth. This was different. Not only did I have those out-of-whack hormones that confused the hell out of your body—particularly with a C-section, when one minute your body is pregnant and the next it is not—but my mind took a while to catch up to the physiological stuff. So, I had all of that working against me combined with the torture of not seeing my own kids. It was an invitation-only event, a one-person pity party of heartbreak.

Those other mothers got to fall asleep skin-to-skin—post-birth—with their babies on their bare chest. They got to snuggle them, hold them in their arms and breathe them in. They got to change that first poopy diaper with the black tar-like meconium. They got to attempt the glory that is breastfeeding. They got to snap endless selfies and family pictures to send out to their family and friends. They got to proudly share their baby's stats—such as height and weight—bragging as if it was a college acceptance letter. I couldn't do any of those things. All I could do was sit and wait some more until those drill sergeants told me I could go up the NICU and see my babies.

There was a faint knock on the door. The curtain slid open, and there was Ed with my parents and Abby. I wasn't sure if they would allow me visitors because they wanted me to "rest," but this was the most amazing gift to me. Abby started to climb up onto the bed with me and cried, "Mama!" I leaned in and kissed her cheeks. "I want my Mama," she said sweetly.

"I missed you, baby girl, I'm happy you are here." I held her tightly as a tear trickled down my cheek.

She was wearing one of her favorite summer dresses—white with navy-blue stripes and little strawberries all over. Her hair was parted down the middle and tied into two little pigtails with a tiny red bow. I couldn't help but think what a hot mess I probably looked. My hair was wildly out of control. I still had my hospital bracelets on—the ones that held my identification, which they told me would match Katie and Lauren's bracelets. The cannula that was attached to the IV to keep me hydrated was stuck to the back of my hand, and I was still catheterized. I must have looked a fright. But in the eyes of your twenty-three-month-old, you are first and most importantly her mother.

"Mama, what's dat?" Abby said, pointing to the IV. I twisted my arm to show her.

"It's a little tube that gives Mommy some medicine," I said.

"Mama, are you sick?" she asked, beginning to lift up her dress to expose her belly—a nervous habit I had noticed in the months before I left for the hospital.

"No baby, don't worry. Mommy is okay."

"Where are shisters?" Abby asked pointing to my belly, which had shrunken in size.

"Abby," I paused and then turned her face towards mine. "Sisters, Katie and Lauren were born today. The doctors helped get them out of Mommy's belly. They are in their nursery upstairs."

"I wanna see! Do they have toys for me to play with, Mama?" her face lit up with excitement. She was remembering the toy bin hospital services had brought, but they'd cleared them from my room, maybe because they had expected me to be going home. Nope. I was still there.

Her expression was so joyful. I couldn't do it. I couldn't be the one to break the news to Abby that she was not going to be able to go up to the NICU to meet her sisters. The NICU had strict policies on who was allowed there. Understandably, they wanted to protect their little patients. I wouldn't want someone else's germy kids near my little preemies. But it broke my heart that she wouldn't get to meet her sisters until they came home, whenever that might be.

This journey had been difficult for us all, especially Abby. I could only imagine what had been going through her little mind through this process. Where's Mommy? Where's my house? When can I go play with my friends? To have to be kept from your mother—even temporarily—is a concept difficult for a child to understand, especially one so young. It brought me comfort to know that she had spent her days happy with her grandparents and had grown attached to Papa. Being just shy of two, she would most likely not remember any of this. That was also reassuring. She would grow up one day and have our family and friends tell her about the pregnancy journey we all went on through. I'd get to share the song I wrote for her, "Together Again," and she would be old enough to understand it. Know the lyrics by heart, even. One day, this would all be a distant memory. Or at least I hoped it would.

"How do you feel, *mija*?" My dad leaned in and kissed my forehead. He was wearing the green shirt I'd given him for Christmas, tucked in neatly. His hair was combed to the side, the way he wore it on Sunday mornings when we went to church.

My mom came over and sat on the other side of me and embraced me tightly.

"We were so worried," her voice was cracking, "we're so glad you are okay." Tears rolled down her cheeks.

My dad handed her a tissue and put his arms around us both. My parents seemed older to me. Stress and worry seemed to have piled on more wrinkles and gray hairs. At that moment, I was so thankful to have them both with me in my room. Thank goodness they didn't feel the need to dramatize things more than they already were. I didn't know if I could have handled another round of, "Oh my god you almost died, the babies almost died." We sat together, holding onto one another. Our moment was interrupted by a soft knock on the door.

"Come in," I said, wondering who it could be.

In walked a young doctor maybe in his mid-twenties. I didn't recognize him. He had green eyes and short, sandy-blonde hair that was combed to the side. He held my medical file in his hands. I could spot the Duffy name.

"Hey, Crystal." He shot me a warm smile. "I'm Dr. Watkins, a senior resident in the NICU. I have some updates for you on your daughters, Katherine and Lauren."

"Oh, yes!" I said, and sat up straight, pulling my hair behind my ears. I'm sure my hair was still a big mess and my face was probably red and splotchy from crying. I reached for a tissue on my nightstand and wiped my runny eyes and nose.

"Mama," Abby said pulling on my robe. "I want a snack."

"Come to Papa," my dad said as he pulled Abby into his arms.

"We will take Abby to the cafeteria so you and Ed can talk to the doctor. I'll call you later," my mom said as they made their way to the door.

I had been wanting an update on the girls since I had woken up in the recovery room. How were they? Did they come out breathing on their own? Did they have to be intubated? But my eagerness was tempered by nervousness. They had kicked Ed out of the room hours before, so I didn't know what I was about to hear.

Ed slid into the spot next to me where Abby had been, grabbed my hand and kissed the back of it. "I love you," he mouthed silently.

"I'm going to start by saying congratulations, you two, for welcoming these two little girls into the world," the doctor said.

This sounded like the same spiel he must give to all new parents when he made his rounds. He looked like just a kid. Was he even old enough to be our doctor? Did he pass his board exams? Qualified or not, he was warm and had a calming bedside manner. After the day I'd had, I was grateful for that too.

"Let me share their birth stats. Katherine (Baby A) weighs three pounds, two ounces, and is fifteen-and-a-half inches long. Little sister Lauren—by about twenty seconds," he laughed cheesily, "weighs three pounds, one ounce, and is also fifteen-and-a-half inches long."

My heart lit with excitement to hear their names spoken out loud. To most people, three pounds would seem tiny, a preemie, as they are known in the medical world. But to me, three pounds was huge. It was a monumental birthweight. I had held them in my belly safely eight weeks past the diagnosis of twin to twin. At the time of the ablation surgery, they had barely weighed over a pound, and now here they were weighing slightly over three pounds. Good job, Mama.

"Katie was breathing on her own when she was born," the doctor continued, "but the NICU nurses put her on CPAP so she wouldn't distress." I had remembered what CPAP was from my preemie book. It stood for Continuous Positive Airway Pressure and was a particular type of breathing therapy. Basically, it was a little mask they put over the baby's nose to constantly blow air. The constant pressure encouraged open airways and reminded the babies to breathe again.

"Lauren was intubated with a ventilator because she was having a little more trouble breathing. We are predicting, though, that by tomorrow she will join Katie and be put on CPAP as well." He nodded, looked back at his notes and continued.

"Both girls had good Apgar scores." He looked pleased, like a professor assessing student scores on an exam. I vaguely remembered this from my reading—methods used to summarize the health of a newborn baby. Assessing their Appearance, Pulse, Activity and Respiration. Oh, shoot I couldn't remember what the G stood for. I made a note in my phone to Google it later.

"They were both started on IV fluids to increase their blood glucose." He paused a moment to let me catch up. I'd swiped a pad and paper from my nightstand drawer and was frantically writing everything that came out of his mouth. I needed to know everything the doctor was talking about. This was a life and death situation. I had to understand every measure that was being taken to help aid my girls' growth.

"Each baby in the NICU has a team made up of an attending, a resident and two nurses. Your babies each have their own team. We made the decision to put them on antibiotics for precautionary measures, and they are being administered ampicillin and gentamicin. And while their blood count is good, we are a little worried about something."

He paused and bit his lip. My hand was still scribbling everything down fast, as my brain struggled to catch up to what he had just said.

And then, it did. Worried, did he just say worried? Oh goodness, what now? "Sorry," I said, "can you repeat that last bit, Dr. Watkins?"

"The nurses noticed some bloody stool in both girls, so we ordered an ultrasound," he explained. "While looking closer on the machine, we noticed that there is a significant amount of blood in both the girls' lungs, in particular, Lauren."

"What?" I exclaimed. "How did they get blood in their lungs? Did it have something to do with the twin to twin disease?"

"When your placenta abrupted, you bled so much that the girls swallowed the blood in utero. It's a miracle they were delivered when they were. Any longer and…" He stopped without finishing his sentence.

"Any longer and what, Dr. Watkins?" Ed snapped.

"When babies swallow that much blood, they go into a state of shock. So, shortly after Katie and Lauren were born, our teams assessed the situation. That's when we realized the girls had swallowed around eight ounces of blood, and we had to act quickly and pump as much as we could out of their stomachs. That's why your husband was asked to step out of the room for a minute."

I started tearing up again. "Is this something that will work itself out, or will they need to have a corrective surgery? What's next?"

"It's something that myself and the other attendings will continue to monitor closely—we expect to get more bloody stools, and perhaps some residuals when we start their feeding."

"Residuals?" I asked. I was unfamiliar with the term.

"It basically means they will probably throw up a little blood in their feeding tubes. Again, it's something we will monitor. If it doesn't clear up in a few days, we will call for a gastro-intestinal consult. Considering everything they went through, they are doing great." And then he smiled his contagious smile. "They're little fighters—it's that kind of strength that helps babies thrive in the NICU and gets them home sooner."

I was relieved to finally hear a good piece of news. I had strong faith in my girls. They were little fighters and—remembering all the fierce ninja kicks in my stomach—I smiled as I imagined their feisty firecracker personalities lighting up the NICU.

"I'll let you guys get some rest." Dr. Watkins said, and then he turned to look directly at me and Ed. "I know it's been a long and difficult day for you both. Please feel free to call me if you think of any questions."

He smiled again, shook our hands, and handed us a card with his phone number on it. And he walked out the door.

The consult with Dr. Watkins had brought me comfort and peace. Maybe not everyone in the NICU was a general. They were trying to take care of our babies the best they possibly could. I was still frustrated and disappointed that I couldn't be with my babies, and still chained to my hospital bed. Only now, it was an IV and a catheter that was keeping me there, rather than 24/7 fetal heartbeat monitoring.

My stomach was numb and if delivery of Abby was any indication, would probably remain numb for the next twenty-four hours, at which point I'd receive a less potent dose of painkillers and the pain would gradually set in. But hopefully, by that point, they would let me go up to the NICU and I'd be able to see the babies. I was eagerly awaiting tomorrow morning. After a long and draining day, all that mattered was that I had delivered my babies safely. They were stable, and now I was able to move onto my next objective: getting them home.

WAITING

I have deep admiration for all the nurses who took care of me during my long stay at the hospital, but the team that took care of me the night after the C-section had the tallest order of any of them. It wasn't because of the high-risk or Mono-Mono twin pregnancy. The amount of blood that had to be wiped, the gauzes that had to be changed—any person without clinical background would run—the nurses dealt with it so calmly and efficiently. Despite being well looked after, the physical discomfort was intense, and I was not able to sleep well. My insomnia was compounded by concerns about Katie and Lauren. Unlike with Abby, there would be no bassinet next to my bed, no late-night stargazing snuggles.

I awoke groggily the next morning. The breakfast tray had been brought into my room, I moved it aside and reached for the water cup. I chugged the whole cup down. I looked for the phone receiver next to my bed and pressed "O." I heard Jenny's voice on the other end of the receiver.

"Oh Crystal," she said, "I'm gone for a couple of days, and I missed all the excitement. Hang on." She must have dropped the receiver on her end. She dashed into my room.

"I missed your birth," she said sounding disappointed.

"I know," I said, "but you are here now."

She walked over to me and I threw my arms around her. I hugged her tightly and began to sob uncontrollably. I cried because I was in so much physical pain, I cried because I was heartbroken leaving my babies upstairs and I cried because of all those damn hormones. I needed the tears to cleanse myself of some of the pain I'd experienced; I feared the next round of it. How was I going to leave my babies in the hospital when I was finally discharged? What if something happened when I wasn't there?

After a few minutes, when I finally loosened my arms and let her go, I opened my mouth. I tried to say something, but the words didn't come out.

"I'm here for you, sweetie," Jenny said, "whatever you need. I'm going to put a 'Do Not Disturb' sign on the door. You don't need people coming in and out for the slightest nonsense," she said, stroking my hair.

I tried again. "I need…" My voice trailed off. "A pump," I finally whispered.

"Oh yes, your milk should be coming in," Jenny said. "I'll call down to Lactation and have them bring you the pump."

"I can take care of that," said Ed, who had been standing at the door, patiently waiting to see what he could possibly do to help.

"You get some rest now, honey," Jenny said and switched off the lights. Ed helped me to lie on my side.

"I'm going to go grab some coffee, I'll be back in a little bit," he said; he flung the curtains and closed the door behind him. I was alone in my room. Alone in my thoughts. Alone to cry. And I did. I cried until I was all dried up and exhausted. I cried myself into a deep sleep.

I woke up to the faint sound of a voice. It was Jenny's.

"Dr. Cooper is here to see you, honey." She leaned over and touched my forehead. "Oh no, you are burning up. Let me grab the thermometer." As she ran out the door, I saw that Ed and Dr. Cooper were on either side of the bed.

"When can I go up and see the babies?" I said.

"Crystal, you are not going to be happy with me," Dr. Cooper said, "but it's looking like the day after tomorrow. Assuming everything stays on track."

I was shocked. I couldn't believe he wasn't clearing me right then and there.

"What? I can't go up there now?"

"You have a fever of 101," he said, looking contrite. "I'm sorry, kiddo. We need to focus on you—getting your strength back and getting you healthy. You lost a lot of blood; that was no small surgery you just had. If by tomorrow night you're in good shape, fever-free, you will be able to go up to the NICU the next day."

Now I was really pissed. Seriously? Why was it so difficult for a mother to be with her newborn babies?

I kept myself as busy as I could the rest of the day and into the next morning by pumping my breast milk. I was diligent about pumping. I set my alarm for every two-and-a-half hours and pumped for at least fifteen minutes—depending how much would come out. At first it was very little—like five to ten milliliters—then it started to increase to several ounces. Every drop I pumped was liquid gold, a commodity so valuable that only a mother could produce it. I was convinced that, even though I was trapped in my room, I was still helping my babies. I collected every last drop of that milk and emptied it into the sterilized containers the lactation consultant had brought me. I neatly labeled every container—as the NICU required—with the date, amount and my name. The NICU had a gigantic freezer to store all my milk. The girls would be bottle-fed with my breast milk. There would be no need to supplement with formula since I had enough milk to feed the entire nursery of infants. I was damn proud of my milk production. My family jokingly nicknamed me Elsie, the cow from Borden's milk, which I never took offense to, since in this case, it was an accomplishment. Over the weekend, Ed frequently visited the NICU and checked on the girls, bringing me updates on their progress and showing me pictures and videos he had taken. The pictures and videos had been huge for me since it allowed me to see the girls and stimulated my breasts to let down the milk.

"Look," Ed said, "here's one of Katie with her little sunglasses on for phototherapy." He smiled proudly as he held up his phone for me to see. "This is helping treat their jaundice." Each treatment was one step closer to the girls' release.

Finally, two painfully long days later, I was cleared to head up to the NICU. Ed had continued to spend the nights with me at the hospital. "Just like old times," we joked. My sister-in-law Bridget had been a godsend and moved into our house temporarily to help take care of Abby. We spent our usual Sunday nights together, ordered take-out and watched *Game of Thrones* on the iPad. I was so excited that the next morning I'd finally be able to go see the girls.

I woke early, as I always do when I'm excited about something. The time I'd spent resting, hydrating and eating over the previous two days had been great for me. I was able to bounce back from this C-section faster than my first. I'm sure it had to do with my determination to get up to the NICU. I threw on a pair of yoga pants, my "Twin Mom" tank top that Ed had bought me as a gift and grabbed a sweater just in case it was chilly in there. It was liberating to be out of that damn bed, without the assistance of a wheelchair and walking on my own two feet.

We navigated out of the labyrinth of the antepartum unit, made our way to the elevator and up to the seventh floor. Our hospital was known for the having a level four NICU—the highest level of NICU in existence. I knew my babies were in the safe hands of trained and caring people. I had gone on a tour of the NICU before the girls were born. But returning there to see my babies would be emotional, beautiful and complicated all at the same time.

"Slow down, Crys," Ed said as I power-walked through the long corridor after the reception desk. I reached the white door at the end of the hallway with the little lamb mascot on the outside. I took a deep breath, turned the handle and stepped inside.

THE NICU

There were bright fluorescent lights overhead, and alarms were going off like fire engines. The room was full of medical staff and machines. There were six other beds in our room, but I didn't hear a single cry or whimper. There weren't any other parents or family members around, just doctors and nurses scurrying around. It was so loud in there. I didn't know how I would ever be able to get used to that. *How could babies sleep through that?* I wondered. And then I saw them.

My daughters were enclosed in massive incubators surrounded by plexiglass, like Snow White. They were wrapped in wires and IVs with big monitors beside them to track their heart and oxygen rates. There was one set tubes helping them breathe and another set checking their heart rate. There were little adhesive stickers all over them to keep the wires in place. There was a tiny pulse ox wrapped around the feet, and it shined a red light through the skin. I would later learn that this little bracelet measured the amount of oxygen in the blood. I would become familiar with all the terminology as if I was the neonatologist. But in that moment, I was the mama expert, and that was plenty for me. I took a deep breath and looked past all the medical equipment and just saw the beauty of our two miracle babies. I was in awe of their survival and how, at just three pounds, they had entered the world triumphantly. They were survivors, they were fighters and they were ours.

Ed and I had gone through a thorough sterilizing process so we would be able to touch them. I insisted on soap and water even though the nurse that greeted us at the door said the hand sanitizer was sufficient enough. They were too delicate to be held; I knew that much already. A young nurse in her mid-twenties approached us. She had long brown hair that was pulled up in a ponytail and wore glasses. Her scrubs were rainbow colored, a design Abby would have loved. She introduced herself, but moments later I forgot what she had said her name was. My strong desire to be near my babies was interfering with my comprehension of basic information. I wished I would have kindly told her, "Can you just give us a couple of minutes? This is my first time meeting my babies." *I know you have a lot of information for me, but please just let me take this in,* I thought.

"The babies have a team assigned to them, who rounds twice a day to discuss updates and a plan of action, etc."

Shhh… I told her silently. *Let me have this moment. This moment I've been dreaming about since the moment Dr. Cooper told me I was having twins. This moment Ed and I had prayed for countless times since we had first learned of the complications. This moment that is finally here.*

We hadn't really discussed which one of us would meet which baby first, so it sort of just happened naturally. I took another deep breath and braced myself, then stepped up closer to the incubators. The Duffy twins' incubators were placed side by side with the monitors in the middle. Ed went to Lauren's incubator and I made my way to Katie's. The incubators had been decorated by my friends—the antepartum nurses from the fifth floor. There was a colorful little poster that said, "Welcome Baby, Katie. Love your antepartum family." There was a soft pink giraffe lovie placed on top of her incubator. I wiped a tear that began to trickle down the corner of me eye.

I rubbed my hands with sanitizer again and slowly opened the little window on the side of the incubator. I was nervous to put both hands in at once because the more windows you opened in the incubator, the colder it would get inside, and I didn't want her temperature to drop.

It was nice and toasty inside her crib, like someone was baking a loaf of bread. Her bed was padded and cushy, and molded to try and imitate the inside of my womb. I moved my hand slowly towards Katie. She was the tiniest little baby I had ever seen in my life, but her skin felt warm and soft. How long had I wondered, hoped and prayed to have the chance to meet her? The experience was surreal. I gently rubbed her back and touched the top of her teeny tiny diaper. It looked like it would fit one of Abby's dolls. Where do you even buy diapers that small?

I touched the edge of the wrinkly little feet that were curled beneath her. She had a head full of tiny black hairs. Maybe Katie and Lauren would look like me and not the spitting image of Ed, like Abby. Her skin was translucent and so incredibly soft. I couldn't tear my eyes away from her. I was in love again in that instant, just as I had been with newborn Abby. The circumstances were completely different, but that bone deep, unconditional love, that connection, that strong bond—it was all there. When I'd examined every little detail on Katie, I turned and looked at Lauren.

"Katie is on C-Pap and Lauren is too, right?" I turned to ask the nurse. It was a different nurse with us now. She was middle-aged with wavy blonde hair, and there were little lambs all over her bright purple scrubs. She had her name tag front and center where I could see her name was Lily.

"Yes, Lauren was intubated yesterday but we put her on C-PAP today." She answered and looked down at their medical charts. "They are doing great. They have a little bit of a feisty personality though, your girls, eh?" She chuckled.

"Yes ma'am," Ed replied. "These two are strong and feisty, just like their mama." He winked at me.

"I have no doubt they are going to do great in the NICU," she said as she looked at their monitors.

That prompted the question Ed and I had been eagerly waiting to ask.

"Lily, do you know approximately how long they will have to stay here?" I blurted.

"Well it's hard to say because every baby—or in your case babies—is different. You can double-check with the doctors when they do their rounds, but we usually tell parents to plan for your baby to come home around their original due date, maybe a bit longer depending the circumstances."

"Oh wow, okay." I said, disappointed. "We have a full two months to go. My original due date was August 24." We were barely in mid-June, which meant they'd be there through the hottest time of year.

"The babies may surprise you and come home early," Lily said sweetly.

"Wouldn't that be amazing?" I said. "Nothing in this journey has been easy or quick."

"I know, I'm so sorry." The nurse shook her head sympathetically.

"I'm here to help your babies and to help you both in any way I can. Basically, babies have to meet three criteria in order to be discharged from the NICU," she said, holding up three fingers to count them off.

"They have to be able to breathe on their own, regulate their own body temperature and be able to feed effectively, steadily gaining weight."

I turned and looked back at the girls; they were asleep. "Okay so we have a little way to go," I said, "but we will get there."

"And no desats for five days in a row," Lily added. "So, technically four things."

"What's that," I asked.

"A desat or desaturation is the decrease in the amount of oxygen in a baby's red blood cells. It's serious and I've seen it really frustrate families when their babies are so close to getting discharged and then the baby will desat on day four and we have to start back at the beginning."

"Oh no, that's awful."

Lily explained to us all the housekeeping and rules of the NICU, she told me I could call at any time, day or night, to check on our babies. She told us about the Ronald McDonald house and how it was a place solely for parents—to eat, drink or even spend the night in one of the rooms. She even told us some places to grab food in the hospital that were better than the cafeteria food. There was an overwhelming amount of information. I had a good memory for recalling details and facts, but given the past few months, my brain had maxed out and was on sabbatical. I hoped it would come back soon and help me navigate through this strange new place.

Ed and I connected eyes and gestured that we wanted to switch babies. I walked slowly to Lauren's incubator, watching my path carefully so I wouldn't trip over a cord. I approached the plexiglass and peeked in, and to my shock and surprise, she was awake. She was lying on her back, her arms folded up and her hands bent near her head. Her tiny little legs were making little kicks in the air. *Oh yes, I remember those,* I thought as I rubbed my stomach. I missed feeling them inside me. And then I looked closer, and she shot me a crooked smile.

"Oh, my goodness," I said loudly. Lily and another nurse turned to look in our direction. My heart was palpitating.

"Ed, get over here, she's awake!" I shouted.

"Look at that," he said with a huge grin. "Well, hello, Lauren."

Lily walked back over to the incubator.

"She must have heard your voice and recognized it," she said, smiling.

"Thank you, thank you, baby girl," I told her. "You have given me the greatest gift. I didn't know how I was going to be able to leave you here. I still don't know, but that smile and your awareness of my presence out here has given me a boost of strength."

And then, in a low, crooning voice, I sang Lauren the song I'd written for her and her sister.

So many times when I thought of you
I worried for your life that you'd be okay
I prayed that you'd come to me, safely
I always remained strong in my faith
And knew that the good Lord would deliver you

Into my arms sweet baby of mine
It was only just a matter of time

I'm singing this to you now
And I'll sing it again when you're in my arms
There has never been anyone just like you
You're amazing, unique, and beautiful too
I love you my darling, I'll always be with you

When we are together just the two of us
For that one moment in time
Everything else in the whole wide world, pauses
And we are the only ones that remain

I'm singing this to you now
And I'll sing it again when you're in my arms
There has never been anyone just like you
You're amazing, unique, and beautiful too
I love you my darling, I'll always be with you

CHAPTER 27

THE LONG GOODBYE

For another four days, we continued our routine. I would rest in my room for most of the day but make my daily visits up to the NICU. The woman at the front desk where the sign-in sheets were placed began to recognize me and call me by name. She would call back to the nurses to let them know I was coming in. Each morning around 7:00 a.m. the residents and attendings would round on their patients. I quickly learned the schedule and tried to be present as they briefed each other on Katie and Lauren's progress. Though it often seemed that, no matter how hard I tried to be there, I would always just miss them.

A week had gone by since the birth and the day that I had looked forward to for so long had finally come—I was being discharged. I'd been in the hospital thirty-eight days and I felt like a lioness being released back into the wild after being held in captivity. I had longed to be able to walk out the front doors of the hospital, look up at the sky, feel the warm summer breeze in my hair and drive anywhere I wanted. At many points during my stay, I would've floored it eighty mph out on Interstate 10 if I could have. But now, that feeling had changed. I knew that, when I walked out those sliding doors, I would be leaving a huge part of myself at the hospital. Katie and Lauren would be under the full care of someone else, not their mother. I would've gladly given back the keys to freedom if it meant I could've stayed with them longer.

On the day I was discharged, I looked around at the walls that had been my home for those five weeks for one final time. My stash of snacks had all been eaten, my clothes had been packed away in my suitcase and my countdown calendar had been taken down, along with the photos of Ed and Abby. A small gray travel bag containing the rental pump and equipment were the only things left next to my bed. All that was left to do was sign the discharge papers and say goodbye. I didn't have the courage to do what I had to do. How was I going to leave them? My thoughts were interrupted by a familiar voice coming in from the hallway. It was Dr. Cooper, dressed in real clothes instead of his usual blue scrubs or white lab coat. His khakis were tan-colored, crisp and perfectly ironed. His shirt was starched white, and his hair had been combed to the side. I almost didn't recognize him.

"Hey, kiddo, today is the day," he said, cheerily. "Are you ready to go home?"

"I'm all packed up, if that's what you mean," I said. "But I'm not ready to leave my babies. Can you extend my stay?"

I buried my face in my hands. He came over and gently rubbed my back.

"Crystal, you've been through a lot," he said. "You were here a long time and you gave birth to two little girls who need you to go home now, get some rest and come visit them when you can."

He gave me a side hug. "Do you get what I'm saying? Don't beat yourself up—I know you feel sad about leaving, but this is just the next step on this journey."

I used my finger to wipe the corners of my eyes and leaned over the nightstand to grab a tissue.

"Thank you, Dr. Cooper," I looked up at him with my weepy eyes, "for everything you did for us—for my family."

"You are very welcome," he said. "It was an honor and pleasure to have gone along on this journey with you. I'll see you in a couple of weeks for your post-op checkup. So rest up." He was very emotional; I'd never seen him show the slightest trace of emotion before.

I nodded my head in agreement. "Of course. So, Are you going to church?" I joked, pointing to his clothes.

He laughed. "No, I'm actually headed to their airport. I'm going to my cousin's wedding in New York. But I wanted to check on you before I left."

He was a brilliant, talented—and might I add life-saving—doctor. He hadn't left my side the whole time. He even brought me snacks on weekends after his family had gone shopping at Costco. I was his high-risk patient, the one that had probably kept him from traveling anywhere that summer.

"Dr. Cooper, you did good."

He opened the door, then turned back to me.

"No, we did good," he said.

A few minutes later, Jenny walked into my room holding my discharge papers. I was glad she was there for my last day as a patient. It seemed only fitting—she was the one who had checked me in, and now she was the one signing me out.

"All right, shug," she said, "I just need your autograph in a couple of places, and you are a free woman. Is Ed on his way?"

"Yes." I looked down at my cell phone. He had just sent me a text message saying he was parking.

"How do you feel?"

"Jenny," I told her. "On the one hand, I can't wait to bust out of these doors, sleep in my own bed, be at home with Ed and Abby again, but on the other hand, the mere thought of leaving my babies behind is too painful to think about, let alone have to do."

"Oh, honey—" She was cut off mid-sentence by the sound of her pager.

"Hang on, someone is paging me. I'll be right back." She darted out the door.

I got up and went into the bathroom, dried my eyes off with a tissue and put on mascara and lip gloss. I came out of the bathroom, sat on the window bench and just stared out the window.

"All right, are you ready to break out of here?" Ed said. He had quietly come in and walked towards me. "Someone is very happy Mommy is coming home today."

"Ed," I said, turning to face him, "I can't do this. I can't abandon my babies. I just can't."

"Crys," he said as he sat down on the bench next to me, "I know this sucks. I hate it as much as you do. But you know what—this may seem like the hardest thing we have had to go through, but it's not." He paused and wiped the beginnings of a tear from the corner of his eye. "Getting the initial twin to twin diagnosis was much worse." We both nodded in agreement. "We're in the clear now, we just have to get through a few tough months."

"Yeah," I said. "As much as this majorly sucks, it's reassuring to have them outside of my body where we can keep a close eye on them. Those machines, they will let us know that they're okay."

There was a knock on the door.

It was Dr. Miller.

"Hi Duffys!"

Ed extended his arm to Dr. Miller. I stood up from the window bench, walked toward him and gave him a hug.

"How are you Crystal? I heard you were going home today so I wanted to come by and say goodbye."

"I wish I was staying. Dr. Miller can you find a way to keep me here?" I asked.

"Oh my dear, I know this is so difficult, but look at how far the girls have come. The worst is over for them. You guys, you've got this," he said sweetly.

My tear filled eyes looked into his piercing blue ones. I gave him another hug and whispered, "Thank you."

My emotional state didn't allow me to adequately articulate into words how thankful and grateful I was for him. The man who had once terrified me had helped us defeat the deadly diagnosis. And now, whether he knew it or not, had become a part of our family's lives forever.

"I have something for you." Dr. Miller said.

He reached into his white lab coat and pulled out a card from his pocket.

"I know it may be too soon for you guys, but I would love for you to join us at the Fetal Center reunion in a few weeks. It's one of the best parts of my job to be able to see all the families, my former patients. It's wonderful to see how everyone is doing."

"That's wonderful. We will do our best to make it Dr. Miller. Thank you for thinking of us." I said.

There was another knock on the door.

Susan popped her head in, and behind her were Caroline, Paul, Ashley and a few of the other nurses I'd come to know throughout my stay.

"We wanted to come say goodbye," Susan said.

We said goodbye to Dr. Miller and greeted our new visitors.

"We're usually so happy to see our long-term patients go, but you are an exception—we wish we could keep you. We all feel honored to have been on this journey along with you. We brought a few gifts," Susan said.

She approached me with her arms full of toys.

"Oh, you guys are so sweet. You didn't have to get me anything." I could feel tears starting to surge.

Caroline came up and gave me a side hug.

"Susan got some toys for the girls—two pink giraffes for Katie and Lauren, and a Doc McStuffins doll for Abby. I recorded your songs "Together Again" and "Never Been Anyone Just Like You" on CDs so you can play them for the girls, and here's a copy of all the love songs that we played the night of your anniversary in the conference room."

Paul came over and hugged me. "Crystal, I will miss you, gossip sessions and junk food chow downs. Now I won't have anyone to discuss the *Real Housewives* with," he laughed. "But you know, I will think about you always, anytime I come down to this corner of the pod. Room 582. It will forever be the Duffy girl room."

Yup, and now full-blown waterworks. *Y'all are killing me here*, I thought, wiping my eyes. Ashley came over.

"Crystal, we are kindred spirits, you and I. Thank you for opening up to me during our many ultrasound sessions. Your girls are lucky to have you as a mother. I will miss you, I consider you a friend. I got you some things too." She handed me a pink gift bag. "I think you'll find these things soothing—some essentials oils, lavender to relax you, candles and lotion." She hugged me tightly.

I wanted to tell them they were like family and let them know what they meant to me—that I couldn't have survived the past couples of months without them. But the words just couldn't come out. Tears rolled down my cheeks and I couldn't let the words escape. Here's what I wish I would've told them.

To Susan—thank you for being a mom to me in the hospital. Thank you for our romantic anniversary surprise in the conference room, it's an anniversary we will never forget. Your love, kindness and positive encouragement is something I will never forget either.

To Caroline—thank you for helping me write and put to music two beautiful songs about my girls. It was a cathartic process that will always be meaningful to us. I wish you all the happiness and success in the world. One day I know you will make a great mom.

Paul—thank you for coming by daily, eating junk food and watching reality TV with me. Your jokes made me laugh during my moments of fear and anxiety.

Ashley—my beloved ultrasound technician, who I'd come to know so well especially in the weeks leading up to Katie and Lauren's birth.

You were like a guardian angel for my girls. You spoke up and reported a finding that we could have easily overlooked. You went above and beyond the calls of duty just to advocate for my babies' safety. For that, I will never forget you.

There were no words but we did several rounds of hugs; tissue boxes were passed around since we were all crying up a storm.

As I stopped to blow my nose, I realized Jenny was not back yet. Where was she?

"Crys," Ed turned to me, "we really need to get going, especially if we are going to stop by the NICU too."

I sighed with disappointment. "I can't leave without saying goodbye to Jenny."

"I'll go get her," Susan said and she darted off towards the nurses' station.

"Let me take your things to the car, and then I'll come back," Ed said. "That should definitely give you enough time to wait and say goodbye." Ed picked up my rental breast pump, grabbed my purse and left the room.

The group slowly started dispersing, each apologizing for having to get back to work.

The last person with me was Ashley, who stayed until she had to go for a scheduled ultrasound.

"I plan on going up to the NICU frequently and visiting the girls," she told me. "I feel like I know them, having stared at them on a screen for two months."

She gave me one last hug and walked off. I looked back down at my cell phone: twenty minutes had come and gone and Jenny still hadn't returned. Ed would be back any minute and would insist we get going so that we could have enough time with the girls in the NICU.

I could just imagine him saying, "You can visit her on one of your return visits to the NICU." Then Ed appeared in the hallway.

"Okay, you ready to go, babe? I called for a wheelchair on my way up, and they should be here any minute."

I didn't want a damn wheelchair. I didn't want to leave the hospital. And I certainly didn't want to leave without saying goodbye in person to Jenny. She had become such a big part of my life in those weeks. She was the person I called when I needed anything—be it glass of cranberry juice or help getting out of the shower. She was the one I had confided in during my deepest, darkest moments of fear and uncertainty. She had also confided in me, trusted me. I knew she would miss me too, and I just couldn't leave without saying goodbye to her.

"Okay Crys, the wheelchair is here," Ed said as a young male volunteer in a red vest appeared around the corner, pushing a wheelchair.

I slowly sat in the chair, and the guy pulled the foot rest down for my feet. It was too late, and I didn't feel like arguing with Ed. I'd used up my last chance to see Jenny one final time. We started wheeling down the long corridor to the elevators up to the NICU. Ed pushed the elevator button. As the doors opened up, I heard a voice scream my name from down the hall.

"Wait, Crystal!" Jenny was running towards us.

"Get me out of this damn chair." I hollered and struggled to stand.

"Oh, honey." She was red and out of breath. "I was afraid I missed you. That IV took forever." She paused and looked down at her shoes.

"I don't even know how quite to put this into words," her voice started to break and she was still trying to catch her breath. "It's always hard to say goodbye to long-term patients. You get used to having them here, you get attached to them. I'm so happy for you, for the birth of your beautiful baby girls, for surviving this place. And for having gone through everything you did. I'm going to miss you so incredibly much."

She hugged me.

"I'm honored to have been your nurse, to have met you, to have gained your friendship, and to have been part of this incredible journey with you."

I was full-on sobbing as she reached into her pocket and pulled out a tiny white box tied with a pink bow.

"I got you a little something."

"Oh, Jenny," I said through my tears, "you didn't have to get me anything."

"Open it," she said. I untied the bow and took off the top. Inside was a long silver chain link necklace decorated with five little charms—each a different colored stone.

"This is beautiful." I said wiping my eyes.

"There's an initial charm with a letter on the front, one for each of your girls. A for Abby, K for Katie and L for Lauren. And these two other stones represent the babies you lost. The birthstone is the month that they would've been born. I thought it was a beautiful way to show your history of motherhood."

"Jenny," I said, struggling to get it together enough to speak some words. "This is the most meaningful gift I've ever received. I will think of you always when I wear it, my dear friend."

I wrapped my arms around her and gave her one last, deep hug. As I slowly sat back down in the wheelchair, I became full-on hysterical. "I don't want to leave! I'm not ready to leave! You can't make me. I don't want to leave my babies!"

What was I going to do without my hospital family? They had been there for me every day for the past five weeks. I never expected that saying goodbye to this family would be as painful as it was.

"I promise to keep in touch, Jenny," I told her. "I will never ever forget you."

Jenny smiled and nodded. She was waving goodbye.

Ed rubbed my back and grabbed the chair's handles and started pushing me. I was still sobbing uncontrollably. People we passed in the hallway were staring. I didn't care.

We reach the NICU door and stepped inside. And just like that, the sorrow of saying goodbye to the people who had cared for me gave way to guilt about the goodbyes I would soon be saying to my own babies. We were greeted by Lily and another young nurse.

"Hi Lily, how are the girls doing today?" Ed asked.

"Hi Mr. and Mrs. Duffy," Lily replied. "They are doing well. Their weight is steady and there haven't been any residuals for the last two feeds. That's a great sign that their little GI systems are getting better."

I got up from the wheelchair and walked over to Katie. My eyes were puffy and everything was a bit blurry from all the crying. I put my hand on the plexiglass and peeked in. She was fast asleep on her stomach.

"My little Katie, I can barely get the words out, my precious love," I told her. "I got discharged today, I'm going home." I paused, my voice breaking. "Please know that you are not alone. Your sister is here with you. I will be back to see you tomorrow, I promise."

"Crys, honey," Ed said putting his arm around my back.

"Just back off, Ed," I said loudly and pushed him away. The nurses stopped their conversations and looked at me. The other families in the NICU were watching too. I went to Lauren's incubator.

"My little Lauren." My words were barely comprehensible. *I'm a train wreck*, I thought. "I'm not abandoning you, my love, I'm going home, but I'll be back tomorrow. I can't wait. Please take care of each other, my precious girls."

I fell to my knees, crying, my arms clutching the side of the incubator. And then I screamed, "I DON'T WANT TO LEAVE MY BABIES."

"All right, I'm taking you home, sweetie. You need to rest," Ed said as he picked me up off the floor and steered me to the door. Lily followed us into the hallway and helped Ed get me into the wheelchair.

"Thanks, Lily," Ed said. "It's just heart breaking for Crystal, leaving her babies. It's not just that they're in the NICU, it's everything. We've been through a lot."

"I know, Mr. Duffy, please don't worry about us. We understand, and we will take excellent care of Katie and Lauren, Mrs. Duffy," she said, reaching for my hand.

"If you want, you can call the NICU office tonight and the nurse on duty can give you an update on the girls."

"Thanks, we'll definitely call later," Ed said as he slowly wheeled me down the hallway.

I left my heart in that NICU room. My babies were no longer inside of me, nor were they in my arms; they were in that noisy, chaotic room inside a pair of plastic boxes.

CHAPTER 28

HOME BITTERSWEET HOME

Ed wheeled me through the glass doors of the hospital.
I was free. The sun was shining down on me and the warm summer breeze collected my hair. It felt so good to be out. Ed steered the wheelchair towards the valet and handed the attendant his keys.

"I'm so ready to be home," I said as I squeezed Ed's hand.

"I know, and you will be very soon."

I hadn't noticed that the attendant pulled up a minivan right in front of us. *Wait this isn't our car,* I thought.

"Surprise!" Ed said as he reached his arms out, pointing to the minivan. It was brand-new and light blue—the sun was shining down strong on it, making it reflect like a mirror—but I could see the big pink bow on the hood.

"What, are you serious?" my face lit up with excitement. *Was this my push present?* I thought.

It was the minivan we had decided on together all those months ago—before any of this—the minivan we wanted to upgrade to for driving our family around. We'd decided on it just a couple months after we found out we were having twins. We'd made a visit to the car dealership one pretty afternoon in February, which is generally a pretty cold month in most parts of the country, but Houston February days are often crisp, clear and sunny. I had insisted on test-driving every single type of large SUV or minivan so I could pick the one that was best for us. Well—me, really, since I would be the one driving the girls around. "This is the one," I said, happily bouncing up and down in the driver's seat of the big, blue, less-than-sexy van. "It drives less like a school bus." Ed must have made a mental note and filed it away, but we had been so wrapped up with this pregnancy that the thought never crossed my mind again. I had assumed we would return to the dealership the weekend before the girls were released from the NICU—whenever that would be—as one of the last-minute pieces of preparation for their arrival.

I had exited the hospital doors heartbroken. Never would I have thought something like a minivan could have impacted me the way it did. But it was more than just a minivan, it was Ed's thoughtfulness. He had taken the initiative to get us the minivan we would be picking up the rest of our family in, and that meant so much to me. Plus, he'd realized that the last thing I would ever want to do after the hospital stay would be to go sit at the car dealership again. Ed told me that his dad had done most of the work in getting the minivan—talking to the cars salesman, negotiating all the discounts and getting everything ready, while watching Abby as she played around the showroom floor. Ed and his parents were able to straighten the whole thing out in just a day to make sure it was ready.

I was so glad to at least have that one weight lifted. This minivan was also a huge assurance that Ed was going to help me make this transition back home. He was going to be there with me every step of the way, just as he had been in the days, months and years before. As I slid into the front seat of the minivan beside him, I knew things would soon be okay again.

Ed turned the key and unlocked our front door. We went inside our house. The time I had been away had felt like an eternity. But, in an instant, the familiarity returned to me—the squeakiness of the door when it was closed shut, the creaky sound the wood floor made when you stepped on it, the smell of fresh pine from the boughs we kept in a vase on the dining room table. I remembered it all.

I heard the pitter-patter of little footsteps running towards me.

"Mommy!" Abby came running to me with her arms stretched over her head, signaling me to pick her up. I carefully sat on the floor and let her climb into my lap. Bridget had fixed her hair in pigtails and dressed her in little pink doctor scrubs that she had gotten for her as a big girl gift. She looked adorable—it felt so good to hug her. I wrapped my arms around her little body, kissed her cheeks, twirled her curls around my finger and put my head against hers.

"Welcome home, Crys," Bridget said to me as she bent down and gave me a hug.

"Let me run and get your stuff out of the minivan. I'll be right back," Ed said.

"I can help you, Ed," Bridget said as she got up and followed her brother. I loved that Ed took his time outside, in the Texas summer heat, to let me and Abby have a few moments alone. I had waited and dreamed about this moment countless times in the hospital as I cried myself to sleep. I was finally back together with my precious Abby. I had missed her so much that there were moments when I wondered if a mother could die from the longing to be with her child. I couldn't wait to play her the recording of the song I had written for her. Would she remember it from the hospital? Would she fully understand the lyrics? Probably not at that point, but one day she would. Completely against my recovery instructions, I picked her up and held her tightly, trying to make up for the lost time when I had been without her.

CHAPTER 29

IN MY ARMS

For the first night in a month-and-a-half, I was able to sleep without being poked or prodded or woken up hourly by a machine's alarm. That said, I didn't sleep particularly well. I woke up in the middle of the night gasping for air. It was too dark and quiet, I had grown used to the light pouring into my room from the hallway and the distant chatter of my nurses at all hours of the night. I would turn to lie on my side and I would feel phantom kicks. I missed the girl's movement inside my belly as much as I'm sure they missed being inside of my body.

I was still in the process of weaning myself off painkillers. While they were helpful to get me to drift off to sleep, I woke up to pump every couple of hours. The overpowering guilt of not spending every waking moment in the NICU caused me to go into milk-producing overdrive. I would fill ten to twelve ounces in just one twelve- to fifteen-minute pump session. In the insomnia that came from the post-pumping session, I thought about Katie and Lauren, alone in their incubators without their mother and without one another. I must have called the NICU eight times that first night.

Abby being home with me soothed my guilt-stricken soul. At moments where I felt a breakdown beginning to emerge, she would come into my room and ask me to play with her or just want to be near me. Bridget continued to stay with us and helped me at mealtimes and bath time. At night, we put Abby in our bed even though Ed was nervous about her rolling onto my still-healing stomach. I had tossed the green folder with discharge and recovery instructions from the hospital in the trash. I was re-writing my own version of the healing process and it was working for me.

Of course, the hardest part of being at home with Abby meant it was hard for me to leave her during the day to go to the NICU. I was done saying goodbye to her, so the next morning Ed and I left early, before she was awake. He dropped me off at the front of the hospital near the valet and arranged for a wheelchair to help me while he parked the car. The wheelchair wasn't for me, but to carry the haul of milk I had pumped the previous evening and other goodies I had brought for the girls, including matching onesies and little pink crochet shoes that my mom had made for them. I took the elevator up to the seventh floor and walked towards the reception desk to sign in. On the sign-in sheet in bold letters were printed the words "visitor."

"Sign your name right there on the line," the receptionist said to me.

But I'm not a visitor, I thought. *I'm a parent and I'm here to see my children. Shouldn't this say plainly parent and child? I should have my own badge to get into the unit instead of being buzzed in like a delivery boy.*

I went through the double doors and walked back to our girls' pod, the sheep pod. I walked past the nurses' station and saw Lily.

"Hi Mrs. Duffy," she said.

"It's okay Lily, you can call me Crystal," I said, smiling.

"Okay great," she replied, smiling back. "I have some wonderful news for you."

My heart skipped a beat.

"I can bring my girls home today?" I joked.

"Ha, not quite. I was advocating for you and your husband during rounds this morning. I mentioned how I really trusted you, even from our first interaction, I got a sense of what warm, gentle and loving people you both are. Usually, with babies this medically fragile, we wait a couple more weeks before allowing the parents to hold their babies, but we think y'all will do great." She paused. "So you can hold the girls today."

"Are you sure? Oh my goodness, that's amazing," I said practically jumping up and down. "I'm sorry for my meltdown yesterday, it's just that being discharged and leaving Katie and Lauren—it was just too much."

"Oh please, don't apologize. I'm so sorry you have to go through this. I know this has to be probably the worst thing you've experienced. But I promise to take care of your babies as if they were my own. That's how I am with all my babies."

"Thank you, Lily. That means so much to me."

"Okay, let me grab you some gowns," Lily said. She walked over to the linen closet and pulled out two bright yellow, polyester, full-length gowns.

"We really recommend skin-to-skin with your babies. There's a bathroom right outside the door if you want to change in there." She pointed outside the room. "You can take off your shirt and have the gown open in the front."

I turned to exit the pod and ran into Ed.

"Is everything okay? Where are you going?" He asked.

"To take off my shirt so I can hold our girls." I smiled.

"I like your "Twin Dad" shirt, Mr. Duffy." Lily said.

"Oh thanks, I wore my *Star Wars* "Twin Dad" t-shirt today to show the girls," he smiled sweetly.

We exited the pod, a few minutes later we both walked back in with the gown over us.

"All set then," Lily said. "Preference to which baby you hold? And sorry, you can only hold one baby each today. We don't want to stress them by having them outside the incubators for too long."

"Oh, right." I was disappointed, but grateful that the team had voted in favor of us holding the girls.

"I'll hold Lauren," I said, "since I spent most of the time with Katie on my first visit."

It felt strange and unnatural to have to ask permission to hold our babies. I had to just keep reminding myself that we had two medically fragile little miracle babies. The nursing team were their primary caregivers right now, and their job was to advocate for their health, safety and protection. While I was still the mom, I was not calling the shots here.

I leaned back in the wooden glider. It reminded me of the one my Ita had in her house from when she rocked her babies. I scooted right up against the incubator. My gown was open in the front, the top of my chest exposed. Lily pumped some hand sanitizer into her hands and then handed the bottle to me.

"I know you washed your hands when you arrived but just being cautious," she said.

"No problem." I replied and rubbed the gel into my hands. Lily unlatched the door and slowly opened the side of the incubator. She placed her arms over Lauren, it looked like she was adjusting something. She paused for a moment before she slid her arms under Lauren, carefully navigating through all the wires that were on her. She had her central IV and then the wires administering nutrients to her, and the ones checking her heart and temperature. Instantly, I became overwhelmed with the sight of all the wires, second guessing my ability to hold my own baby. Was I really qualified for this? But before I could say anything Lily was holding Lauren right in front of me.

"Mama, here's Lauren," she said, slowly placing her on my chest. Then she wrapped my gown around her like a blanket. She turned and bent down to open the lower drawer under the incubator and pulled out a tiny little crocheted hat.

"I'm going to put this on her head so her temperature doesn't drop." It looked like a baby doll hat that had been weaved together with tiny, sparkling silver strands.

"That is precious," I gushed.

"Aren't they? They were donated by some of our nurses as little gifts for our preemies."

Man, I wish I could sew, knit or really do anything domestic, I thought.

"Lauren, it's Mommy. I'm here sweetie. I love you."

I'd imagined every detail of this moment for months. How I would feel, what my babies would look like and the amount of love that would beam from me. The moment took my breath away and I just sat there in silence breathing in my baby. I caressed her fine, black, silky hair and held her tight against my chest. Here little legs barely extended to the top of my bra. There was a strap that held her ventilator tube in place; it covered most of her face and there was a heart-shaped sticky pad that held the wires on her chest. None of it mattered to me. She was beautiful, tiny and perfect. And she was in my arms.

I watched Lily as she walked over to Katie. She opened the side latch and then slowly opened up the door on the side of the incubator. She placed her hands slightly over Katie's chest, at first glance I thought she was going to adjust the wires, but then I saw her close her eyes and whisper something. She was saying a prayer for Katie. A prayer of hope, a prayer of love, a prayer to guide her—to heal in whatever way necessary. She scooped Katie up in her arms and turned towards Ed who was sitting in his glider.

"Here's your little angel, Daddy," she said as she placed Katie on his bare chest.

There was a deep love and connection that our nurse Lily had for her babies. The way I imagined all NICU nurses have for their baby patients. At work, they care for the babies as if they were their own and truly empathize with the mothers. Some may have had a NICU experience themselves, while others had worked around these medically fragile babies enough to understand how the parents felt when no one else—family, friends, everyone—could. I knew Lily understood the pain I felt leaving the hospital without my babies. She knew how heart-wrenching it was for me to be away. She knew that we were experiencing the darkest, most difficult time in our life, and all she was trying to do was make it a little easier for us. For the first time since I was discharged, I was at peace knowing that, while I wasn't able to stay at the hospital 24/7, when I left I would be leaving my babies with their angel caregivers, the NICU nurses. And for that, I was so grateful.

CHAPTER 30

FIVE WEEKS

It was a complicated monster of a feeling that engulfed
me over the next few weeks. There was the calmness, relaxation and joy
I got just from being in my own home and being with Abby. Getting to be
her minute-by-minute mommy again brought me back to my balance
and moved me away from the hysterical mother who'd left her babies
in the NICU. This huge pleasure, however, was counter-balanced with
a deep sense of guilt. It was similar to first-time mommy guilt—the kind
you get with things like sleep training or leaving your baby at school for
the first time, only multiplied by a hundred. I felt like I was abandoning
my babies because I didn't spend every waking moment there at the
hospital. No matter where I was—my house, my parent's house, the
grocery store, anywhere besides the NICU—this feeling occupied my
every thought. Even when I was there, as I pumped, waited, worried,
held them, and then pumped some more, I still felt guilty because I'd
left Abby. I had left her for months already, and every day when I got
dressed to "go to work," meaning spending the day in the NICU, my
heart broke all over again. I was stuck in a horrible cycle of leaving one
to be with the other. It felt like complete and utter agony, and no matter
how many times Ed, family and friends told me not to beat myself up, I
still continued to.

On one Saturday afternoon in late June, my parents were grilling
outside in their backyard and had invited us over for lunch and to go
swimming. I got through half of the meal and then turned to look at Ed.

"You want to go see the girls?" he asked me.

"Yes, very much so." I said.

We excused ourselves and I wrapped up my hamburger in a napkin to eat in the car; we drove the hour to the hospital from my parents' house.

Throughout the months of June and July, my world revolved around Kangaroo care, bilirubin lights, surfactant, residuals, reflux and poop-inducing glycerin drops. It was monumental to us when the nurses informed us, about a week-and-a-half after the girls had arrived, that Katie and Lauren were being transferred out of the danger zone and into the intermediate care unit known as the feeders and growers floor. The room looked more like a hotel than a hospital—it was a private room with a view of the zoo, incubators placed side-by-side like they were college roommates, a private bathroom with shower and even a fold-out bed for parents to crash on. I never imagined after I was discharged that I would want to spend even one more night in that hospital. But the excruciating pain of leaving my tiny babies up there in a room all by themselves pulled me (and often Ed) to stay there for hours into the night and to eventually pass out on the pull-out couch. On those nights, I slept peacefully being with my girls, surrounded by the beeps and alarms of the monitors—a sound I'd gotten used to.

On the days I slept at home, I would wake up, have breakfast with Abby and then pack my work bag—as I called it—for the day. It held all the gear I needed to pump—the bottles, the printed labels from the NICU so I could identify which baby they were for, a hands-free pumping bra and some snacks/lunch and plenty of water for myself.

I loved being there first thing in the morning—when the babies woke up and were very alert and smiling—it made for the best snuggle time. I would hold the girls. In the beginning, I held them one at a time, but after I got more comfortable, I would ask to hold them together. I read the girls books, Abby's favorites from home, sang them songs, and rubbed their backs.

Back when we were in the danger zone floor, Lily had explained to me the three-hour feeding routine. It started at 6:00 a.m., then 9:00 a.m., then 12:00 p.m. and so on throughout the day. One morning I woke up very early around 5:00 a.m. and couldn't fall back asleep. I left Bridget a note that I was leaving for the NICU. I hurried and drove through morning rush hour traffic across town so I could make it by 6:00 a.m. and do the girls' feeding myself. I walked into the girls' room at 5:55 a.m. and saw that the nurse on duty had already fed them.

"I thought the feeding was at 6:00 a.m.?" I said out of breath from my brisk walk over from the parking lot.

"It is. I just did it a little early so I could get ready for shift change," she said. "The nurse shift change is at 7:00 a.m. and you will have to step out of the room," she informed me. "Why don't you go and grab some breakfast and come back after the shift change. You can hold your babies then."

I said nothing. I turned and ran down the hallway. There was no one in the Ronald McDonald house, I went in and threw my bag down on the floor. I plopped down at a table covered in oatmeal packs and pretzel bags and wept. I was torn between my two worlds. I had missed everything. I didn't get to have breakfast with Abby at home, nor did I get to feed my babies breakfast at the hospital. I left the hospital a little early that day to spend the afternoon with Abby. We watched movies and went out for ice cream.

Ed and I celebrated huge milestones—the kind you don't read about in *What to Expect When You're Expecting*—like being able to hold the girls together at the same time for longer than just a few minutes. We were ecstatic the day Katie and Lauren transitioned from a feeding tube to a bottle—we rejoiced that they were able to keep down just a few cc's of breastmilk at a time. I was overjoyed when there were no more tubes or cords taped to their skin or their little tiny faces. We could finally see our babies without any medical devices obstructing our view. We could finally touch and caress their soft skin and kiss their noses and cheeks.

I was elated when we could finally start dressing them in clothes other than the NICU-provided onesies and could buy them tiny little outfits.

Ed and I marveled at not just every ounce of weight the girls gained, but at every gram—the unit of measurement that they used for preemies.

"That's all you, Crys, your breastmilk," Ed told me with a smile.

My body had not only known that I was having twins, but that they were little preemies who needed to grow, and I would need to supply them with as much nutrients as possible. And I did. And for that I was very proud.

One day, Ed and I walked into the girls' room and saw that they had been moved from the incubator into open-air cribs. They were growing, approaching 1600 grams, a milestone which was no small feat. The babies were nothing short of miracles. Each day, they continued to amaze us with their strength and perseverance—and their love for food. As happy as I was that they were thriving, it still didn't ameliorate the emotional rollercoaster we were on. As we left the day we'd seen the girls in open-air cribs, I started to cry. We had had such a beautiful afternoon of laughs and giggles and photo snapping, but it could not take away the throbbing ache that came from having to leave your children behind. It was too much. As we drove home in the car, I erupted into tears.

"What's wrong sweetie," Ed asked. "We had a great visit."

"WHAT's WRONG? WHAT's WRONG?" I yelled. "What's wrong is that we are here—driving home, and our babies are there, stuck in that room, alone. And I don't know when that will ever change!"

I ended up driving back to the hospital again that day. I wanted to visit Jenny, Ashley and Susan on the antepartum floor. As I waited at the front desk for Susan to come and greet me, I watched her come through the double doors and into the waiting area. I could tell right away that something was wrong. I suspected that it must have been a rough day—maybe a patient hadn't been as lucky as me and suffered a miscarriage.

"Is everything okay?" I asked.

"Crystal, I'm so glad to see you. I just got some terrible news."

Just then, Jenny came through the doors, also looking very upset.

I didn't know what to think or say, so I just listened.

"There's no easy way to say this," Susan said, "but something terrible and shocking has happened to Ashley." She dropped her head.

"Ashley, my ultrasound tech?" I said. "Is she sick? What's wrong? Has she gone back to California?"

Jenny and Susan exchanged a glance. "She passed away on Tuesday morning," Susan said.

WHAT? Wait, What? I thought. *This is not real. That can't have actually happened!*

"How?" I screamed. "I don't understand, what happened?"

"She missed work Monday and didn't call or message anyone. Everyone assumed she was sick or just forgot to notify us she would be absent and didn't think much of it. When she didn't come in on Tuesday, people began to worry because that was very unlike her. Someone finally got a hold of a friend of hers and they went over to her apartment. They found her. She died in her bed."

"I still don't understand," I said. "Was she sick?"

"She had been out sick last week with the flu. She had an auto-immune disease, and her body just was not able to recover."

"I can't believe this." I put my head in my hands, still working hard to process this shocking news.

Ashley, the ultrasound tech I had gotten to know so well. For five weeks, I had seen her almost every day. She was the one who always saw the girls and told me what they were up to—what position they were in. She was the one who had notified the doctors of all the fluid at the last biophysical ultrasound scan. That was the Friday before they were born. We would have never known they were in potential danger if it hadn't been for her. I couldn't believe she was gone.

Susan and Jenny stayed with me for a while in Susan's office. We talked, I cried—still having those excessive hormones. But I was shocked and deeply saddened over the news. She was an excellent sonographer and a true asset to her profession with a wonderful zest for life. She was not even forty; she wasn't married and didn't have children. But she was a daughter and granddaughter. Her family was all in Louisiana, which was where the services were held. I wanted to go so badly. I wanted to be there and hug her parents and tell them how wonderful their daughter was. How she had been my babies' guardian angel on earth. And now she was a guardian angel in heaven. Until we meet again, dear friend.[6]

As I walked toward the elevator, I reflected on how lucky I was that my girls were going to be okay. Every day, people die everything from long-term illnesses to freak accidents. Ashley's passing sounded like it was a little of both. I thought about her parents who might have been afraid for a long time that something like this could happen because of her auto-immune illness. It was a reminder that, even though we had survived twin to twin and a placental abruption, the journey of parenthood was really just beginning. I already knew this from having spent two years with Abby, but this reminded me of the worst part of being a parent: the fear that something would happen to one of my girls. It was a fear that would never go away. I held on to Katie and Lauren extra tight when I reached the NICU.

---

6   Ashley Breux, who served as my sonographer through my time in the Fetal Center passed away on March 12, 2015. I have integrated her death earlier in my story.

CHAPTER 31

THEIR ARRIVAL

There are moments in life that are forever ingrained in our heart and memories. I will never forget, Sunday, July 27, 2014—the day that our babies finally came home. Ed had taken a half-day off of work the Friday before. We had lunch together and headed over to the NICU afterwards to spend the rest of the afternoon with Katie and Lauren, taking turns holding each of them. We arrived at their room, As I bent down to pick up Katie, there was a brisk knock on the door. It was Dr. Wong, the girls' main doctor.

"Hi Mr. and Mrs. Duffy," she said as she entered the room. We chit-chatted for a few minutes, and she asked about Abby—how she was doing and if she was ready to be a big sister.

"Abby was born ready to be a big sister," I said with a smile. "She is gentle, calm, loving—she is going to be the perfect big sister to Katie and Lauren." Dr. Wong nodded her head in agreement.

"Well, she will get to help this weekend," she smiled.

"Oh yeah, how so?" I asked, confused.

"I think this weekend they will be ready," she said.

My mind went crazy. Wait a minute, what did you say? Who will be ready?

"Sorry," I said in disbelief. "What do you mean?"

"I will be discharging Katie and Lauren on Sunday, and they will be able to go home then."

It took a few minutes for the news to sink in. I kept thinking that perhaps I had heard her wrong. That she had gotten us mixed up with another family. But after three rounds of clarification, I knew it was really happening much sooner than Ed or I had expected—than we ever imagined feasible.

In those painful weeks after their birth, it had felt like my babies didn't belong to me, that they belonged to the hospital as property. It was like they weren't even my own, and I was borrowing them when I would come visit. *Thanks for letting me hold my own babies.*

But now my Katie and Lauren, my babies not the hospital's, would finally be coming home—where they belonged, where they had always belonged—with Mommy and Daddy. Suddenly, I was—for the first time since before the twin to twin diagnosis—so incredibly happy. It felt like a devastatingly painful problem had been solved, corrected and finally set right. My heart was full of love and joy.

"They are coming home! They are coming home! I can't believe my babies are coming home!" I repeated over and over again.

Dr. Wong explained how the team had come to their final decision about discharging Katie and Lauren. Basically, Katie and Lauren had thrived during their NICU stay, like the champs and fighters they were.

"Both girls have stayed pretty much in sync since they arrived here. They have met all the requirements we typically use as a frame of reference to see if patients are ready to go home." She paused momentarily to look down at her phone which was beeping.

"They have long been breathing on their own without any assistance, and they have been able to regulate their own temperature since we moved them from the incubator into the open-air cribs. The last thing—they are gaining weight and growing at a rate that we are quite pleased with, thanks largely to your wonderful supply of breastmilk. The nurses told me you have over nine hundred bottles of breastmilk stored in our NICU freezer." Her eyebrows were lifted with excitement.

"Make sure you make arrangements to take it all home with you on Sunday, too," she said. "You will definitely want all of that," she smiled. Ah yes, my liquid gold.

I blushed, "Thanks yeah, I have a great supply. I almost forgot that we would need to take all that home."

Where the heck was I going to fit nine hundred bottles of breastmilk? We would need to get a deep freezer, and that would still only store half.

"Thank you so much for everything, Dr. Wong." Ed said, shaking her hand.

"Yes," I agreed. "You and your team have been incredible to Katie and Lauren, ever since they arrived here to the grower and feeder floor." I leaned in to hug her.

"I can't believe we are taking them home this weekend," I said, tearing up.

It was the most amazing feeling in the world to have given birth to two little miracle babies and to finally—after months of worrying for their safety—being able to take them home. To be able to hold them without someone looking over my shoulder. Without looking up at the clock and assessing how many more minutes of cuddle time you would be allotted. To not have to worry about alarms beeping, monitors going off, shift changes, team meetings, or room cleanings. It felt great to be able to lay them down in their own cribs with their own blankets, and monogrammed lovies—to be able to close the door of their nursery. I could give them a bath whenever I wanted to. We'd finally get to introduce them to their sister and see the interactions between the three of them. Most of all, it felt great to not ever have to leave them. We would be done with all of it. I would finally be saying goodbye to this place forever.

If I hadn't made so many good friends in the hospital, I might have never stepped foot in the doors again. Luckily, that was not the case. There were so many emotions flooding my heart—happiness for their departure, sadness reflecting on all the memories that led to that point and overwhelmed with the preparations I still needed to finish. I began to panic—mentally making long list of "to-dos." Being the over-the-top, annoying perfectionist that I am, I wanted everything to be perfect for their arrival. We had been given a wonderful surprise, but now we were going to run and scramble to finish.

I still talked to the babies in my head even though they no longer lived inside my body. Babies, I told them, this is the most amazing news ever. I'm finally going to be able to take you both home. Free at last!

Dr. Wong was heading out the door when she turned back to us.

"One last thing—make sure to bring the girls' car seats up to the NICU for inspection. The girls will also have to pass the car seat test."

"The car seat test?" I asked.

"It's just to make sure the girls are big enough to sit up in the infant car seat. If you have inserts, I would go ahead and bring them. They can help prop up the babies."

Another thing to add to the list of things we'd quickly need to do and buy—two infant car seat inserts. We never used them with Abby; she was so big that there was no need for one. We waited for Dr. Wong to make a clear exit before we gathered our things and made a mad dash to the car.

"Ed, we need to stop at Target and Babies-R-Us on the way home," I told him as our min-van roared out of the hospital parking lot. My elation had started to mix with panic.

My due date had been August 24. The night Katie and Lauren were born, we had met with Dr. Watkins, the first of their many doctors, and he had instructed us to mentally prepare for the girls to be discharged around my initial due date. That was usually how it went. Not this time! My babies were getting released a whole month early. Whoop whoop!

It was only late July. I'd anticipated having another month to get everything ready. It's not that I had procrastinated or anything. It was the whole bedrest for months thing and the busy shuffling back and forth between home and the NICU. I would usually come home late from my visits, then I would pump and collapse into bed. Day after day. I hadn't managed to carve out time for anything else.

On the Saturday before the big day, I spent hours deep-cleaning the house, in particular the nursery. I scrubbed the floors and baseboards, washed the windows and disinfected the crib rails. I washed, folded and put away all of their clothes, most of which we had received at my baby sprinkle, and others as gifts when I was in the hospital. I meticulously organized the smallest details—labeling baskets for diapers, wipes, burp cloths and setting up their hair bow holder. I picked out their coming home outfits: teeny tiny pink smock dresses my mom bought at the hospital boutique shop that came with matching bloomers and bonnets. They would look like little dolls in their matching outfits. I packed our diaper bag with all the essentials—diapers, wipes, an extra change of clothes for the babies and me (you never know) and at the top, I placed the white crocheted blanket my mom had made them.

Afterwards, I was exhausted. I plopped on the couch next to Ed who was up late working in the living room. He was trying to get as much as he could done before the girls got home; he would be taking a few days off to help me. I curled up next to him on the couch, our hands were interlocked.

"I can't believe tomorrow is the day we bring our babies home," I whispered to him.

"I know," he said, turning to smile at me. "This time tomorrow, there will be five of us—six, if you count Charlie—on this couch."

I woke up a few minutes before my alarm. It was still dark out, and our bedroom was freezing with the AC cranked up and the fan blowing on high. I made a dash for the shower and started getting glammed up. I fixed my hair and makeup and even put on a nice dress and actual shoes, not flip flops. There would be photos. Lots of photos documenting this glorious day. Ed woke during my primping and hopped into the shower. I usually had to drag him out of bed, but not that day. The excitement was too big. My parents had offered to drive to the hospital with us and assist with the girls. They'd gather their belongings, and most importantly, help us transport all that breastmilk home. Abby would stay at home with her Auntie Bridget, anxiously awaiting our arrival.

We got to the hospital quickly. It was Sunday and there wasn't much traffic headed to the medical center. I was pleased we had arrived early. I wanted to get this car seat test over and done with, breast milk packed up and loaded and head back home.

Two of Katie and Lauren's nurses were already in their room when we got there. They were each holding a baby, taking their temperatures and reading their blood pressure.

"These are the last vitals that will go in their charts," one of the nurses said as she jotted down their numbers in her chart.

"We're just about done getting everything we need from the babies," the other nurse said. "In just a minute, we will hand them over to you and your husband so you can get them dressed."

I placed my diaper bag on the coffee table and began digging to the middle of the bag where I'd placed their coming home outfits.

"Here, I can help you Crys," my mom said. Dressing Katie and Lauren was a group effort. Ed and my mom put on the bloomers, bonnets and socks. I wanted to be the one to put the dresses on. My dad was snapping as many pictures as he could. The nurses stayed and snapped some of the four of us. Halfway through our photoshoot, there was a knock on the door.

"Come in, I called out."

When no one entered, Ed opened the door. In the middle of the hallway were four wheeling carts loaded with the hundreds of frozen bottles containing the expressed breastmilk I'd spent countless hours pumping over the last month-and-a-half. Someone had stuffed them in large trash bags and placed them on the carts. Thank goodness for that, because they were heavy. My dad and Ed made two trips each down to the car and loaded all the breastmilk bags into the trunk.

At that point, we knew we that needed to head out fast so the milk wouldn't spoil in the car with the summer heat. I went to the nurses' station to say goodbye and found Dr. Wong and about eight nurses gathered around the desk. They were signing cards.

"Hey guys," I interrupted. "Our car is all loaded up. We're ready to go."

Dr. Wong looked up and smiled.

"Before you guys leave, we have a little something for you."

One of the nurses pulled out two little gift baskets from out from behind the desk, each tied with pink and white balloons that had "NICU Graduates" written on them. The baskets were filled with all kinds of goodies—diapers, wipes, creams, hair combs, pacifiers—and there was even a scrapbook filled with pictures that the hospital photographers had taken at each step of their journey. One card was addressed to Katie, the other to Lauren. Each was filled with personal messages the NICU nurses had written them.

"I enjoyed seeing you grow in these weeks I got to work with you. Continue to thrive and make us proud."

"The Duffy sisters are miracles, and I was honored to serve as your nurse."

"We will miss you, please keep in touch and send us pictures." In the middle of each card, a message had been printed:

Everything is different after you experience the NICU.

You never forget the sights and the sounds.

It all becomes a part of you. It changes you forever.

Watching your child fight for survival gives you

new appreciation for life and the value of it.

Your own child is your hero.

I wiped away tears that had started to trickle down my cheek. I looked up and found the group had gathered around me.

"Thank you all so much for your hard work," I told them, "and for taking such wonderful care of my Katie and Lauren—as if they were your own babies. You all have definitely touched my family, and we will never forget you."

I have always been terrible with goodbyes. I love so strong and become so attached to people, that losing even a single individual from my life is hard. I rejoined my parents, Ed and the babies, who were waiting in the hallway.

Dr. Wong and the nurses followed behind me. We did our hugs and goodbyes. Dr. Wong bent down to look at Katie and Lauren.

"You guys passed the car seat test. You are definitely ready to go home." She tapped the cushion pillow behind them. "You'll probably be out of this infant insert in a few weeks."

"Especially if they keep eating and growing at the rate they have been," I laughed.

Ed and I each picked up a car seat, the babies still fast asleep inside. The team had lined up on either side of the hallway to see us off. It felt like we were royalty as we walked down that hallway, babies in our arms, everyone smiling and waving goodbye to us. We reached the end of the hallway, went through the glass doors of the NICU and into the elevator. As we left the elevator and made the final steps to the main hospital doors, everything came flashing back to me—everything that had led to this moment. Paris, the two blue lines, the blood clot, the twin to twin diagnosis, the laser surgery, my first day at the hospital, the anniversary dinner, the blessingway, the birth, the countless trips up the NICU...there had been wonderful parts to this journey, and devastatingly painful parts too. We stopped in front of the doors, and Ed and I put the car seats on the ground side by side as we waited for the valet to bring our car. Both girls were deeply asleep. I bent down, kissed their feet, and whispered, "You were worth it all, my loves."

The parking attendant pulled up with our minivan and Ed and I picked up the babies and placed the car seats gently in the strapped-in bases. I sat in the back seat with them. The car ride to the house felt longer than it had ever been. I kept telling Ed to drive carefully.

Every bump and turn seemed more obvious due to the precious cargo we were transporting. As we rode, I thought about Dr. Cooper, Dr. Miller, Jenny, Susan, Caroline, Paul and Ashley—all the people who had been on this journey and what they had all meant for me. It had taken a community of special individuals to get us to where we were. The two precious babies sitting in the back seat of our minivan were little miracles that had been born healthy and strong because many important factors had fallen into place. It was just like the card the nurses had given us said—their struggle for their life made us appreciate and value them so much more. No matter how much time had gone by (or would go by in years later) I would remember this heightened sense of value.

We arrived at the house and pulled into our driveway. Abby and Bridget were waiting by the window, ready to greet the girls. I kissed Katie and Lauren on their bonnets.

"I'll be right back, my loves," I told them.

I jumped out of the car, ran inside and scooped up Abby in my arms. She had on her bright green "Big Sister" T-shirt, white shorts and her favorite flower sandals. Ed and I had told her that this would be the day she would be meeting her baby sisters for the first time. I hugged her tight and kissed her little cheeks.

"Abby, sweetie," I whispered, "we are about to bring in your sisters, Katie and Lauren."

She smiled. "Yay, shisters!"

Ed and my dad got the babies—still snuggled tight in their car seats—out of the minivan. My mom snapped pictures every step along the way. I waited in the doorway with Abby in my arms—waited to unite my family. This was the moment I'd prayed and hoped for all those months on bedrest in the hospital. I'd waited so long, and it was here.

They set the babies down on the living room floor and we all circled around Katie and Lauren, gazing at every detail. After about two minutes, I bent down and unbuckled the straps of the car seats. I picked up Katie first, held her for a few minutes and then passed her to Ed while I picked up Lauren. We bent down towards Abby, and she kissed the top of their bonnets gently. She then proceeded to pat their backs. Ed and I moved to the couch in the living room, each cuddling a baby. Our families were snapping more pictures on their phones and cameras. Abby jumped in between us, and of course, Charlie didn't want to miss out on the action. He jumped onto the back of the couch and perched there, looking down at us.

Before I knew it, Katie and Lauren started to wake up and began to whimper little newborn cries. It was time for their next feed and we had forgotten the breastmilk in the car. My dad and Bridget hurried outside to unload all the bottles of breastmilk. My mom ran into the kitchen, grabbed some expressed breastmilk I'd pumped earlier that morning, and started making bottles. With the babies crying, Abby giggling at them and Charlie barking at all the chaos, Ed and I turned to look at each other.

"This is a look into the next year of our life," he said.

There was no denying the mayhem that would be our household that next year—the cycle of feedings, burpings, spit-ups, diaper changes, baths, swaddling and rocking to sleep. As I sat there on the couch with my new family of five, I was able to breathe the way I hadn't been able to for almost a year. I knew in those moments of chaos that we had made it to where we were always meant to be.

2018

They splash, giggling hysterically. The sky is slightly overcast; a rainstorm has just ended. The girls, who had been waiting patiently under the pavilion, rush out to the beach.

"Again, again, Daddy."

They are linked up, holding hands, running into the waves just as they break on the shore. The saltwater splashes into their mouths and their feet sink in the wet sand. Their day's adventures have included constructing sandcastles, whale practice and pretending to be mermaids from the *Little Mermaid* with Ed taking the lead role as King Triton. Now, they are expelling their last bit of energy.

We are in Galveston—one of our happy places. We have taken the girls here every summer since Abby was a baby. I'm lying back on a chaise lounge chair, my pink polka dot beach towel drape over its back. I'm wearing my large, striped sun hat, I have an ice-cold Karbach Staycation beer, and the latest Emily Giffin for book club. Our picnic blanket is beside me, covered with a thin layer of sand and beach toys. The girls briefly take a break from their play and come running back to me, slinging wet sand in every direction. They grab their slices of watermelon, bag of Doritos and juice boxes, fighting over who got more snacks. I smile at Ed, who's drying off with a towel. He walks toward me and kisses me, then acts as mediator for the girls.

"It's getting late—shall we head up and get the girls ready for dinner?" he asks me.

"You guys go ahead," I tell him. "I'll pack and be up in a few minutes."

Ed herds the girls and they make their way back to the room.

It is surreal being here with Ed and our three young daughters. I think back to when I had gone to a different beach all those years before. Did it all have to play out the way it did in order to get to where I am now? There are days I still wake up and think it was all a dream. Did that really all happen? Did we survive the high risk twin pregnancy, my near death during childbirth and the NICU?

Katie and Lauren are now four-year-olds. They are healthy, beautiful, hilarious, headstrong, and at times, like all children, frustrating. I can't imagine one without the other. We have gotten to see them grow, and as each day passes, and we see the amazing relationship grow between the two girls. We know we truly are doubly blessed.

It's getting late and the tide is coming in. I dust the sand off my towel and beach bag and gather the rest of the toys, snacks and a pair of flip flops left behind by the girls. And then I run to catch up with my family.

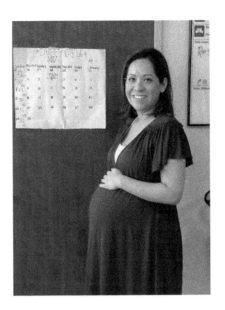

Me, in front of my countdown calendar, marking each day spent in the hospital as a monumental achievement.

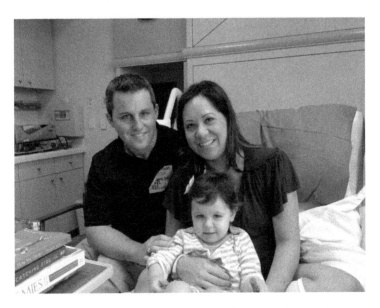

Ed, Abby and me after our hamburger cookout in my hospital room.

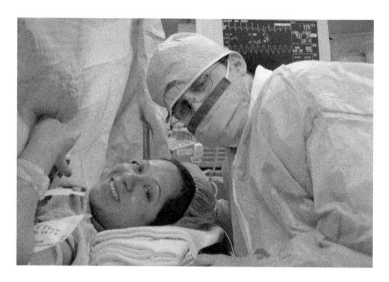

"We are having some babies today!"

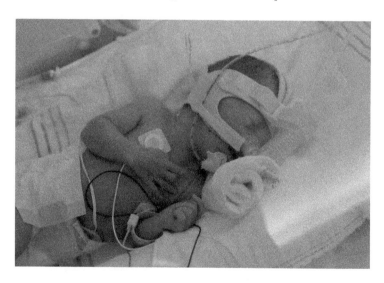

Our first photo of Katherine.

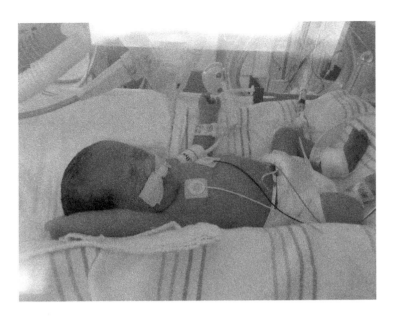

Our first photo of Lauren.

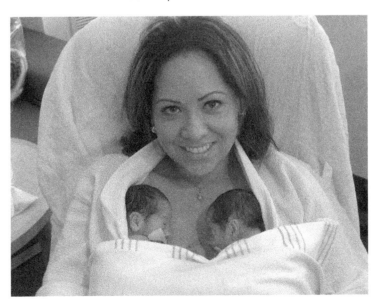

Here I am doing kangaroo care with the girls, a position I would stay in for hours.

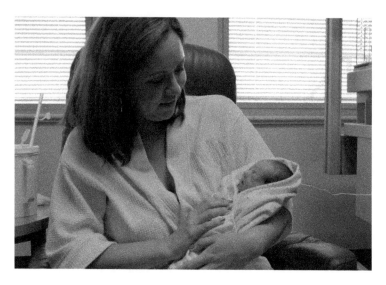

Relishing in every single NICU milestone—we had finally gotten the face tape removed.

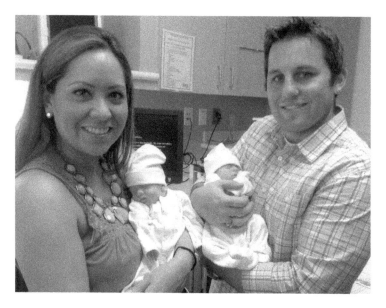

Homecoming day—Ed and I posing for one last photo in the girls' room.

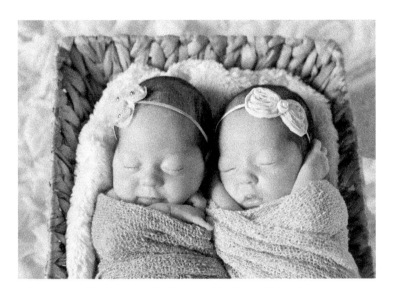

Our newborn photoshoot—Katherine on the left, Lauren on the right.

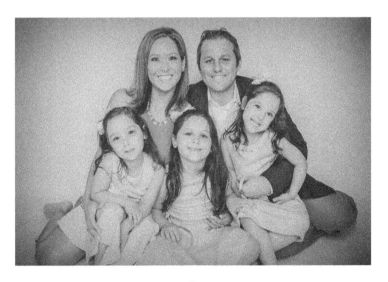

The Duffy gang!

ACKNOWLEDGEMENTS

The process of writing a book and getting it published may actually be more painful than childbirth, even with twins. Well not really, but in all seriousness, a huge thank you to the wonderful people that helped bring this project to fruition:

Thank you to my amazing and hardworking agent and friend, Katie Shea Boutillier, for having confidence in *Twin to Twin* and helping make its publication a reality and for always believing in me. To my amazing editor, Brenda Knight and my talented and amazing team at Mango: Chris, Hannah, Hugo, Ashley, Jermaine, Natasha, Michelle and Christina—thank you for your tireless work in perfecting *Twin to Twin* and getting it ready for publication.

Thank you Dr. Kenneth Moise, a.k.a. Dr. Miller, for the beautifully written foreword—I'm so grateful and honored to have you as a friend, and I am very blessed that you and your team were able to save my girls. Thank you Mark Graham and Ann Tinkham for helping me transform scribbled sleep-deprived written phrases into a story. Tremendous thank you to my blurb writers: Jane Roper, Cea Sunrise Person, Suzy Becker, Marcelle Soviero, Megan Woolsey, Alison Lee, Margaret Welwood and Joan Friedman, Dr. Amir Kahn. Thank you to Mark Malatesta whose guidance and input helped me immensely in my search for an agent. Thank you Susan Krawitz for doctoring my manuscript and helping me strengthen my characters. Thank you Estelle Erasmus for your blurb and for providing invaluable feedback and suggestions along the way.

A special thank you to my Hermann family—Sandra Uribe, Hannah Scott and Lara Lockey—you not only helped my babies make it to delivery, but you helped make my inpatient stay more stress-free and fun than I would have ever thought possible. I would like to remember my angel technician and friend, Ashley Breux, who I wrote about in this book, and who unfortunately did not get to meet my wonderful warriors. Thank you to Dr. Paul Cook for saving my life half-a-dozen times. Thank you to the OB/GYN Centre team—Dr. Melham, Dr. Nanda, and Dr. Papanna—who provided great care to me from the moment

I learned I was pregnant until the girls were safely out into the world. Thank you to my NICU nurses and all the NICU nurses in the world—for the love and care you show all of your babies each and every day. Thank you for helping, supporting and encouraging me—Krysie Webber, Kari Opperman and Andrea Crane. Thank you to my PAC Family—Madelene, Kim, Kitty, Meghann, Kerchalyn, Ashanti, Alissa—who have helped me give back to the community that gave so much to us.

To my big loving Houston family—Justice Eva Guzman, Tony, Melanie, Martha, Spencer, Caroline, Michelle, Stephen, Gregory, Stephen Jr., Andrew, Sandra and Taylor—thank you for always being there for me. To my California/Chicago family—Kathy, Pat, Bridget, Matt, Angela, Jim, Maureen and Eileen—thank you for all your help throughout this pregnancy.

A huge thank you to my mom, Maria, for proofreading my manuscript, for the countless hours of babysitting and for your love, support and faith in me always. Thank you to my dad, Miguel, and my sister Melissa for your endless support and encouragement. Most of all, thank you to my love, Edward, for supporting me always in both in my writing and in life. The best partner to go through this life adventure with me. Thank you Abby, Katie and Laurie, my motivation always. Thank you God, my cup doubly runneth over.

HIGH RISK PREGNANCY AND TWINS/ MULTIPLES RESOURCES

High Risk Pregnancy

Twin-to-Twin Transfusion Syndrome

Twin to Twin Transfusion Syndrome Foundation
http://www.tttsfoundation.org/

Phone Number (24 hours): 1-800-815-9211,

Email: info@tttsfoundation.org

The Twin to Twin Transfusion Syndrome Foundation is the first and only international nonprofit organization solely dedicated to providing immediate and lifesaving educational, emotional and financial support to families, medical professionals and other caregivers before, during and after a diagnosis of twin to twin transfusion syndromes.

Fetal Health Foundation
http://www.fetalhealthfoundation.org

The Fetal Health Foundation provides factual medical information on fetal syndromes, provides unconditional support to families dealing with these syndromes and direct connection to leading fetal treatment centers and doctors around the world. They also provide advocacy and awareness around fetal syndromes and provides research grants funding new treatments and technologies providing hope to save our babies.

Society for Maternal Fetal Medicine
https://www.smfm.org

The Society for Maternal-Fetal-Medicine supports the clinical practice of maternal-fetal medicines by providing education, promoting research and engaging in advocacy to optimize the health of high-risk pregnant women and their babies.

Sidelines—High Risk Pregnancy Support
www.Sidlelines.org

Sidelines is a non-profit organization providing international support for women and their families experiencing complicated pregnancies and premature births.

Heartstrings
http://www.heartstringssupport.org

Heartstrings provides compassionate care, bereavement education and hope to families who have suffered pregnancy or infant loss through distinctive peer-based support programs guided by bereaved parents in partnership with professional facilitators.

Now I Lay Me Down to Sleep
https://www.nowilaymedowntosleep.org

NILMDTS offers the gift of healing, hope and honor to parents experiencing the death of a baby through the overwhelming power of remembrance portraits. Professional-level photographers volunteer their time to conduct an intimate portrait session, capturing the only moments parents spend with their babies. Parents are gifted with delicately retouched heirloom black and white portraits free of charge.

March of Dimes
http://www.marchofdimes.com

March of Dimes fights for the health of all moms and babies. They advocate for policies to protect them and work towards radically improving the health care they receive. They are pioneering to find solutions. Their prematurity campaign works towards research and discovery, care innovation and community engagement, advocacy, education and family-centered newborn intensive care units (NICUs). They empower families with the knowledge and tools to have healthier pregnancies.

Preemie Parent Alliance
http://www.preemieparentalalliance.org/

Preemie Parent Alliance is a network of organizations offering support to families of premature infants. We are the only professional association for NICU Parent Leaders in the United States. PPA provides a platform for NICU Parent Leaders to come together as a collective voice representing the needs and best interests of NICU families in all facets of healthcare policy, care guidelines, advocacy, education, and family support.

Graham's Foundation
http://www.grahamsfoundation.com

Graham's Foundation delivers support, advocacy, and research to improve outcomes for preemies and their families. They provide remembrance care packages as well as peer-to-peer support via email. Phone and text, and have an online community with over 30K engaged parents.

Hand to Hold
https://handtohold.org

Hand to Hold is a national leader in support programs for NICU families. They supply printed educational resources to hospitals to help teach parents how bond with their babies and effectively communicate with their care team. The peer-to-peer support program provides comfort and support to thousands of families each year. They also have a podcast, NICU Now, an audio support series that features insights for medical and mental health professionals as well as NICU graduate parents.

Twins/Multiples Resources

Multiples of America
http://www.multiplesofamerica.org

The Multiples of America non-profit organization dedicated to supporting families of multiple birth children through education and research. Multiples of America promotes, supports and encourages networking for parents of multiples. Opportunities for self-help, emotional support and parenting info are provided through local club and state organization meetings.

Twins and Multiple Births Association (TAMBA)
https://www.tamba.org.uk

TAMBA—Twins and Multiple Births Association—is the UK's leading twins and triplets charity. Packed full of advice and information about what to expect while pregnant, breastfeeding advice and even information about schooling.

Twins Magazine

Twins Magazine is the premiere magazine for parents of multiples, from twins and triplets to quadruplets, quintuplets and more! Published bi-monthly or six times each year, It is the "bible of parenting multiples," loved by moms and dads of twins and high-order multiples since 1984.

Twiniversity
www.Twiniversity.com

Now reaching almost 100,000 families in over 150 countries, Twiniversity is the largest global resource for all things "twinnie." With worldwide recognition in her field, Natalie Diaz brings her twin parenting expertise to an online community where you can connect with thousands of other twin families from around the world. There are also chat forums and thousands of articles written for twin parents.

Twins Doctor
http://www.twinsdoctor.com

Launched in 2007, Twins Doctor is the first physician-authored website to provide health information exclusively for multiples.

Babies in Belly
www.babiesinbelly.com

Babies in Belly offers convenient, virtual prenatal classes taught by a certified teacher and mother of identical twin boys.

Raising Multiples
http://www.raisingmultiples.org

Raising Multiples was founded as MOST: Mothers of Supertwins in 1987 by a community of families, volunteers and professionals. They are leading the national nonprofit provider of support, education and research on higher-order multiple births.

Twin Pregnancy and Beyond
https://www.twin-pregnancy-and-beyond.com

Twin Pregnancy and Beyond was founded in 2007 by a mother of twins on the basis of offering the best and most-up-to-date "twin specific" information and support on all aspects of twins-from finding out about your twin pregnancy, through twin birth, raising twins and beyond.

Twins Day Festival
www.twinsdays.org

The Twins Days Festival is the largest annual gathering of twins and multiples in the world and takes place every August in Twinsburg, Ohio. It's open to twins and multiples of all ages.

Twins Online
www.twinsonline.org.uk

Twins Online is a helpful and informative site loaded with topics covering all aspects of twins.

Centre for the Study of Multiple Birth
www.multiplebirth.com

In 1977, identical twins, Louis and Donald Keith founded this non-profit organization to promote research, education, and public service for multiple births.

Dad's Guide to Twins
www.dadsguidetotwins.com

A Dad's guide to all things twins including finance how to raise healthy babies, tips for physically caring for two, getting twins to sleep and more.

KellyMom
www.kellymom.com

This is one of the most comprehensive websites for moms, and was developed to provide evidence-based information about pregnancy, breastfeeding, health, nutrition and parenting. Kelly is the mother of three children and an International Board Certified Lactation Consultant (IBCLC).

New Mommy Media
www.newmommymedia.com

New Mommy Media is a network of dynamic audio podcasts. Their shows give tips and advice for new parents, education and entertaining moms and dads as they transition into parenthood. Each 30-minute episode features everyday parents and experts discussing relevant issues in a relaxed, roundtable format, and they have a weekly podcast called Twin Talks.

Joan A. Friedman, PhD

Dr. Friedman is a prominent and well-respected twin expert who shares her passionate views and insights about twins and their emotional needs with twins and their families throughout the world. The fact that she is an identical twin and the mother of five, including fraternal twin sons, makes her ideally suited to this task. Her commitment to twin research and her treatment of twins of all ages demonstrate the breadth and depth of her skills and experience.

Multiples Illuminated
http://multiplesilluminated.com

Multiples Illuminated is an online community of twins, triplets and more! Editors Megan Woolsey and Alison Lee birthed their first anthology *Multiples Illuminated: A Collection of Stories and Advice From Parents With Twins, Triplets and More,* featuring essays from *twenty talented writers and parents of multiples.* The second book in the series is now available, Multiples Illuminated: Life with Twins and Triplets, the Toddler to Tween Years.

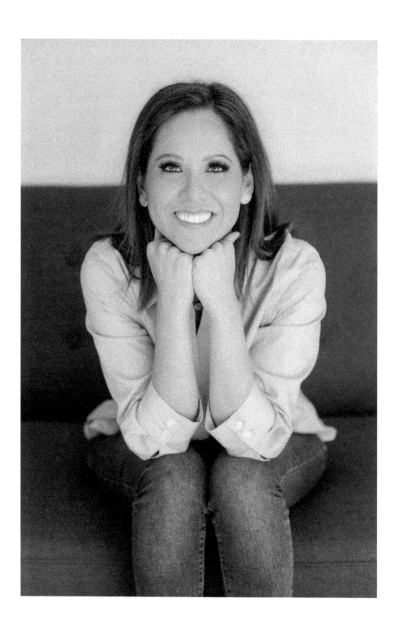

ABOUT THE AUTHOR

Crystal Duffy is a writer, speaker, educator, parent advisor in the NICU, and mother of three little girls, including a set of identical twin girls. She now tours the country inspiring women across the United States recounting her "emotional tale of empowerment." Her essays on family life and parenting have appeared in Woman's World Magazine, Twins Magazine, Scary Mommy, and Twiniversity where she is a senior writer and instructor for an expectant twins class.

Crystal is a graduate of Georgetown University in Washington, DC, where she met her husband Edward. Crystal lives in Houston, Texas, with her husband, three little girls, and a yappy little Yorkie.

CPSIA information can be obtained
at www.ICGtesting.com
Printed in the USA
BVHW031615100219
539889BV00002B/2/P

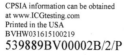

9 781633 538337